OTHER FERTILITY BOOKS BY

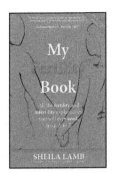

'his comprehensive book explains over 200 complex terms in plain English. Available in print and ebook.

Feeling overwhelmed by the infertility language? Don't have a clue what the abbreviations and acronyms mean on fertility forums, groups and websites? All is made clear in this invaluable resource. Available in print and as a free ebook – download from www.mfsbooks.co.uk

Infertility sucks doesn't it? You shouldn't feel alone whilst on your journey to having a baby. Read real-life experiences and thoughts from the fabulous TTC community, who want to support you and let you know that #youarenotalone. Available in print and as an ebook.

Two weeks of waiting to find out if you're pregnant

#youarenotalone

This is The **Two Week Wait**

Sheila Lamb

Author of the *This is* series

Published in 2019 by MFSBooks.com

Copyright © Sheila Lamb 2019

Cover Illustration Sheila Alexander

Cover Design Marketing Hand

Copy Editor Sherron Mayes, from The Editing Den

Illustrations Sheila Alexander and Phillip Reed

Print ISBN 978-1-9993035-3-2

A CIP catalogue record for this book is available from the British Library

Dedicated to all the amazing women and men who have survived the two-week wait.

This book is intended purely to share people's experiences of trying to conceive and offering words of support.

The information provided must not be used for diagnosing or treating a health problem or disease.

It does not replace the advice and information from your healthcare specialist, such as your doctor, nurse or other health expert. This book does not provide medical advice. The author does not accept liability for readers who choose to self-prescribe.

The information is correct at the time of publication and has been interpreted by the author.

Foreword

I think I officially lost the plot during some of my two-week waits. I became unrecognisable, obsessive, sleepless. I was a woman possessed, living in a parallel universe, where early morning pregnancy tests were positive, and I would wake up my husband, (maniacal heart pumping), with a cup of tea, the coveted two-lines and happy news. Where I would travel into the future, and plan how we tell our families and announce our baby's imminent arrival on social media, with a quirky yet heart-warming image. Where I would buy maternity jeans and take selfies to show off my bump, puffing out my cheeks to match my big baby tummy. Where I would give birth, goddess-like, in a pool surrounded by candles and music. Where we would joke happily about how exhausted we were because the baby didn't sleep, ha-ha. And where I would make birthday cakes and pose for family portraits around a Christmas tree. Oh yes. I spent a disproportionate amount of time in my parallel world compared to the one I was actually inhabiting.

Over time and after many rounds of failed fertility treatment, I realised that living in the future wasn't doing me any favours. I started to throw myself into learning how to do the opposite and remain present, even if the reality was a million miles away from the dream. Because what I had in the real world was just that: real. At least when I stared, empty with despair, at yet another negative pregnancy test and old needles piled in a sharps bin from hormone injections, dreams shattered yet again, I would have something to hold onto that wasn't a dream and was always right there within me: my inner strength.

I found this strength by doing all the things you're told to do. I had such a total turnaround during this self-practiced 'presence work', that about a year later, I started to share it on social media. I thought there must be others who felt like I had. I didn't want anyone else to feel as alone, misunderstood and confused as I had.

It was just around the time that the Instagram TTC community was really kicking off. I discovered thousands of people, all sharing their experiences, connecting in a way that I wish I had found when we were going through our treatments. They were extraordinary. Boosting each other while going through their own versions of fertility hell.

The support and boost to mental well-being that these connections have is truly remarkable. People say it's changing their lives because they don't feel so alone, and they have somewhere to go when they don't know who else to turn to; when the fertility clinic is closed and their best friend unsupportively says "Are you taking supplements? What about putting your legs in the air?".

Sheila Lamb's work on helping to change the narrative and putting together this book is an absolute life saver. She has a knack of putting into words exactly what you feel when you're experiencing a two-week wait, and knows how enormously important it is to surround yourself with people and words which help you cope.

What you'll find in the following pages is packed with funny, relatable, real writing from people who have travelled this path and found ways through it. There's poetry, letters of solidarity and ideas for self-care. I found myself laughing out loud at Amber's contribution (@thepreggerskitchen): "I had squeezed my bloated hippo arse into a new set of knickers, necessitated by ruining all my old comfy ones with progesterone pessaries. An embryo implanting or a tight bit of elastic? It was anyone's guess."

Sheila has collated some of the best writing around on fertility, and put together a fantastic resource for those going through it, and for anyone supporting someone else. I just wish it had been around when I was marooned on my own infertile island with no idea whether I would ever get back to the mainland. This book is your rescue boat - your life raft! Climb aboard and hang on tight. We're not leaving you behind.

What you'll get from reading will be a massive virtual hug from a lot of people who really understand what you're going through. It's like sitting down with your mates and having an honest, open chat; leaving you feeling warm, understood, validated and maybe even with a bit of a spring in your step. Because whatever happens: you are not alone. We've got you.

If you want to join the conversation in real time - come and find us all on social media. There's such a warm welcome waiting for you.

Take really good care, good luck - and whatever happens, you are going to be OK.

Alice Rose x

Fertility Life Raft Podcast

@thisisalicerose

thisisalicerose.com for mindset courses, campaign, blog

catandalice.com live events

Acknowledgements

This book, and the 'This is' series it is part of, would not exist if it wasn't for the women and men who are part of the most amazing and supportive community that ever existed. It wasn't until I joined Instagram after publishing *My Fertility Book – All the Fertility and Infertility Explanations you will ever need, from A to Z*, that I realised what 'community' actually means. Although my rollercoaster journey of four 'two-week wait' periods ended happily several years ago, it has helped me to accept the emotions that come with all areas of infertility, and are still part of me.

My thanks, firstly, go to my miracle, rainbow daughter Jessica, who means the world to me and is my reason for writing and helping the TTC community. This book wouldn't exist if it weren't for the following people who have contributed. Some I have known for many years and met at various fertility events, and others I have only 'met' through the online community. So, in alphabetical order: Alice Rose, Amber Woodward, Amelia Freeman, Andreia Trigo, Anya Sizer, Becky & Matt Kearns, Blair Nelson, Cat Strawbridge, Diane Chandler, Dr Deborah Simmons, Dr Emma Brodzinski, @fertilitysmarts, Gareth James, @herfertilitydiary, @iwannabemamabear, Jackie Figueras, Jessica Hepburn, Justine Bold, Justine Hankin, Kate Davies, Kate @hopematters.always, Lianne Baker, Lisa Attfield, Monica Bivas, @mrskmeaks, Natalie Silverman, Nicola Salmon, Rachel Cathan, Sandra Bateman and Tori Day.

The book cover was illustrated by the author and illustrator, Sheila Alexander, who was so supportive and patient as I stumbled to explain what I wanted for this book and the series. We both, very much hope, you relate to the woman as she plans for her two-week wait, watched by her fur-baby.

Sheila Alexander is the author of *IF: A Memoir of Infertility*, a graphic novel about her infertility treatment using in-vitro fertilization (IVF). She lives in Massachusetts with her husband, son, dog, and parrot. She holds a master's degree in education and is a minor in fine art from Lesley University. By day, she works as a teacher, where she shares her love of comic books with her students. She believes that books have the power to change lives, so she published her first book, in the hope that it would help others who are going through infertility treatments. For more information visit her website: www.sheilaalexanderart. com or follow her on Instagram, @sheilaalexanderart.

Sheila also captured parts of this journey in the illustrations you'll find inside the book, as did the illustrator Phillip Reed, who created the illustrations in *This is Trying to Conceive* and *My Fertility Book*. He can be contacted on info@phillipreed.net and Instagram @phillipreed.

I'd also like to thank the following who have encouraged and supported me to put my *This Is* series of books together: my parents, Paul Lamb, Michelle Starkey, Claudia Sievers, Angie Conlon, Maria Bagao, Judy Marell, Heidi Fitch and Dr Mahadeo Bhide.

Contents

Introduction

If you find yourself reading this book, you have my heartfelt support, because dealing with one two-week wait (commonly abbreviated to TWW or 2WW), is enough for anyone. Or, perhaps you're reading it because someone you care about has gifted it to you, or maybe it was recommended to you, so that you can understand what a two-week wait is and why there needs to a book about it.

Firstly, if you are not quite sure what a TWW is, and there are two kinds, let me elaborate:

1. When a couple decide to try for a baby, most think it will happen the first time they try. After all, in school they were told to be careful not to get pregnant, because it happens so easily. Fast forward fifteen to twenty years, or more, and it's a different picture for some. Around the middle of a woman's menstrual cycle, (this can be a bit vague), she should produce an egg, (not guaranteed), which, if she has sex, (guaranteed), should be fertilised by a sperm, (not guaranteed), which embeds in her womb (again, not guaranteed) and nine months later, a baby is born. When she doesn't get pregnant those first few months, she'll then start to be obsessed with the time between producing an egg and her period, which is roughly two weeks.

2. When the above has been going on for a couple of years, or someone has gone straight to fertility treatment, such as IUI (intra-uterine insemination), or IVF (in-vitro fertilisation), the two-week wait becomes more intense and a dreaded ticking clock. With IUI, sperm is placed inside the womb where hopefully it will find an egg and fertilisation will occur. It's then two weeks until a couple find out if they're pregnant. With IVF, after an embryo (an egg that has been fertilised by a sperm and grown in an incubator for a couple of days), is put into the womb, it's two weeks until a pregnancy test is taken to find out if they are pregnant.

As you can imagine, this is a nerve-wracking period of time. It's bad enough if you have dealt with years of naturally trying to conceive, but when you go down the route of IVF or IUI, it's a whole new level, because so much more is invested in each cycle. Fertility treatments take over your life – there are clinic appointments, blood tests, investigations, scans, injections. But, more importantly, there are the emotions that you can't possibly prepare for, because you don't know how you are going to feel. We are all different and we all deal with things in different ways, but most people dread the TWW because at the end, you either get a positive pregnancy test (possibly the first one ever), or you don't. There is nothing quite like this 336 hours or 20,160 minutes – every hour, minute, second, thinking and wondering if the embryo has stuck to your womb lining and you'll see two pink lines on your pregnancy test.

Finding it challenging to have a baby is a life changing experience for most. It certainly was for me. Even though we were eventually successful, this experience was very much part of my life and what made me, me. Like a lot of people who have a life changing experience, I wanted to give something back to those who also found themselves on this path, to offer help and support. So, I started an online magazine called *My Fertility Specialist* – and the fertility experts who wrote articles, along with the women who shared their real-life stories, were inspirational.

I put together eight issues over two years, and in that time, I started a spreadsheet of all the topics I could utilise for articles and listed them from A to Z. Then I realised that maybe all this information would be better in a book; a jargon-free glossary of all the medical and non-medical terms that people, without a medical degree, could understand in order to steer their journey in the direction they wanted it to take. I put the magazine on hold and concentrated on writing *My Fertility Book: all the fertility and infertility explanations you will ever need, from A to Z,* and published it in 2019.

Most fertility terms have acronyms or are abbreviated, such as AMH, BBT, and 6DP5DT, and are often used on social media, forums, online groups and websites, so I wrote a free eBook called *The Best Fertility Jargon Buster: the most concise A-Z list of fertility abbreviations and acronyms you will ever need.* More information can be found at the front of this book.

Most people don't talk about their struggle to conceive, which also includes the two-week wait, which makes it a very lonely time in their life. They don't share with their nearest and dearest, because they don't want people to feel sorry for them, or worry, but also because they know they might not understand. That's why many people find support and comfort online with strangers who often become friends. Sharing feelings is comforting as you realise that you're not alone, and that it's okay to feel worried, anxious, positive one minute and negative the next. Women and men feel supported, boosted and, most important, understood and validated by a community of other people who also find themselves part of an intimate global group. Nobody wants to be in a group of seeming 'failure to conceive' people, but when you find yourself part of it, boy, they have your back.

It was reading the posts in these communities that gave me the idea of putting all these lovely, warm, supportive, virtual hugging words into a book. Then, if you find during your TWW that it's all getting a bit too insane, reach for this book and read about those who have been there before you, and what they have to say. They'll help get you through it.

Practically all the contributors have experienced at least one two-week wait after infertility treatment, and if they haven't, they have worked with people who have struggled to conceive. They've kindly given up their time to share their own experience for this book. Each quoted extract is in the voice of the contributor.

Remember, there is no right or wrong way to deal with this time, but these inspiring women and men all wanted to share what they did or didn't do, what you should or shouldn't do, in the hope that these words will in some way help you – until you hold your longed-for baby in your arms, and start your lives together as a family.

A letter to someone about to, or going through, a TWW

Dear Friend

Going through a two-week wait (let's shorten that to TWW), whether it's waiting every month or after you've been through fertility treatment, is probably one of the hardest things you will go through. You are not alone – in the UK in 2017/18, there were over 80,000 fertility treatment cycles, so that's 80,000 TWW's, and this figure is similar, or higher, in other countries.

Most of the contributors in this book have had at least one TWW following treatment, and more natural two-week waits than you can shake a pregnancy test stick at. They have written from their heart and share their thoughts and experiences, because they understand how hard it is to deal with this period of time that so much is riding on, and how important having the right support is. We are all much stronger together.

Some words that come to mind about the TWW – dreaded, hateful, scary, torture, agonising, nerve wracking, but also exciting because this could be the cycle that works. We are all different of course, but at least one of the above words will creep into your mind, or vocabulary, during this time. And that is OK and normal. You wouldn't be human if you didn't dread 336 hours of pregnancy mind games:

- What was that I felt in my belly just now, never felt THAT before?

- My little toe itches SO much, could I be…?

- What is it with my boobs today, they are SORE?

- What's THAT? Could it be implantation bleeding?

- How many hours until I can test?

Most of the contributions are from women, but, as men also go through the TTW, a couple have contributed too. Often people forget that their partner is also going through a very hard time – they might not physically be PUPO (pregnant until proven otherwise), but they want a successful outcome as much as the next person. Which brings me onto other people, like family and friends. You may have shared with them my *This is Trying to Conceive* book, so that they understand what it's like to deal with infertility on a daily basis. If you're about to go through fertility treatment, such as IVF, or IUI (intra uterine insemination), you may like to consider giving them this book as well, because trying to explain yourself can be difficult – instead let over thirty contributors tell you about their challenging experiences.

There are a number of ways of finding the support that is right for you, and with every contribution is the person's Instagram handle or their name. If a contributor is someone who helps the infertility community professionally, at the back of the book is a 'Resources' section in case you want to connect with them.

The most important thing to remember is that #youarenotalone in your two-week wait.

Lots of love,

Sheila and the TTC community

A letter to someone who hasn't experienced a two-week wait

Dear Friend,

Firstly, thank you so much for opening this book. It's probably not the sort of book you'd choose, but please read some of it – I think you'll be glad you did. Bear with me while I explain what exactly a 'two-week wait' is.

When a couple are trying for a baby and it's taking longer than they thought, the first thing they'll check is when the woman ovulates, then have sex around that time, and then wait two weeks to find out if she's pregnant. When this doesn't work, as is the case for one in eight couples worldwide, they may try fertility treatments such as medication, IVF (in-vitro fertilisation) or IUI (intra uterine insemination). With IVF, after an embryo (an egg that has been fertilised by a sperm and grown in an incubator for a couple of days), is placed into the womb, there is a two-week wait until they do a pregnancy test to see if they are pregnant. With IUI, the egg is not removed; sperm is placed inside the womb where hopefully fertilisation will occur. Again, there is a two week wait until they find out if they're pregnant. As you can imagine, this is a nerve-wracking period of time.

For a number of reasons, many couples keep the fact that they are struggling to get pregnant to themselves, often because of embarrassment, shame, or that they don't want to worry you. It also isn't an easy thing to talk about. When a couple resort to fertility treatments like IVF, trust me, they didn't make this decision lightly – especially when there are no guarantees that they will get pregnant.

So, I'm sure you can now see that the two-week wait is a very difficult period of time, and you are going to need to be supportive, kind and empathetic. Take your lead from them – if they want to talk about how they are feeling, 'listen', but please don't try and fix anything or say something like: 'It'll be all right' or 'Of course it will be successful'. Remember, there are no guarantees. One minute they'll be hopeful that the treatment has worked, the next, they'll be crying and ranting that they're not sure if they have early pregnancy symptoms or not. Don't be that friend or family member who turns away from someone who needs a hug, or worse, says something insensitive.

You will read about people who have gone through one, or many, two-week waits. Their experiences will help others to know that their feelings and thoughts are perfectly normal at this time. But what we all want is for people like you, who may not have struggled to have a baby – so haven't had to go through fertility treatment, or worry if they are pregnant or not each month – to really understand and hopefully 'get it'.

Although we are all on different journeys to have our much-wanted babies, how we feel is often very much the same. We are a community and we support each other completely. And we hope you get to meet our baby, that we have fought so hard for, very, very soon.

Lots of love,

Sheila and The TTC Community

Imagine if...

You'd only ever been PUPO (pregnant until proven otherwise).

You'd only ever seen one line on your pregnancy test stick.

You'd never seen two pink lines or the words 'Pregnant' on your pregnancy test stick.

You'd never said to yourself in wonder "I'm pregnant!"

You'd never said to your partner "I'm pregnant!"

You'd never heard your partner say "We're pregnant!"

You'd never been able to talk about your unborn baby using their nickname.

You'd never had an ultrasound scan to see your growing embryo.

You'd never heard or seen your baby's heartbeat at the ultrasound scan.

You'd never seen your baby playing hide-n-seek or waving at you at your ultrasound scan.

You'd never made an announcement on social media that you're pregnant.

You'd never felt fluttering movements as your baby moves inside your womb.

You'd never been able to place your partner's hand on your belly to feel your baby move.

You'd never posed for a photo with your hands making a heart shape over your belly.

You'd never sent out invites to your own baby shower.

You'd never get to give your baby the name you and your partner have chosen.

You'd never heard the midwife or doctor say "It's a girl!" or 'It's a boy!"

You'd never kissed your baby's toes.

You'd never felt your baby's soft, downy, warm skin against your skin.

You'd never seen your baby's first smile.

You'd never heard your baby say "Mamma" or "Dadda".

You'd never received your first Mother's Day or Father's Day card.

You'd never heard your baby's giggles as you tickle them.

You'd never seen your baby walk for the first time.

You'd never heard your child say "I love you Mummy" or "I love you Daddy".

You'd never pushed your child on a swing or caught them as they flew down the slide.

You'd never cried at your child's first day at nursery or school.

You'd never held your child's hand as you walk down the street together.

You'd never jumped in muddy puddles with your child or flown a kite.

You'd never built a sandcastle with your child.

You'd never experienced that rush of love you have for your child.

Imagine if you didn't have all your memories of these precious moments with your child or children.

Imagine what it's like for someone struggling to get pregant, so desperate to experience all that you have, and not knowing if they'll ever make these memories.

An impatient girl's tale of an IVF TWW

Let's start off by saying I am the most impatient person on the planet. I do not like waiting five minutes for my latte, much less waiting two entire weeks to find out if I'm pregnant. I also crave answers immediately when I have a question. My personality totally jives with the first part of an IVF (in-vitro fertilization) cycle. It all begins with weeks of frequent appointments, bloodwork, ultrasounds, calls from the doctor to go over results, and extensive feedback on what my body is doing.

With the holy grail of IVF, the embryo transfer day is no different, as you're fussed over and given multiple instructions:

- Wake up at the ass crack of dawn

- Drink water on your way to the office − but never too much

- Check in and suit up - hello gown, my old friend

- Every detail is narrated by the nurse, doctor, embryologist, and all questions answered − are you sure that's our embryo?

- Shimmy from one gurney to another, get in position, catheter inserted and embaby delivered into your womb

- Finally, lay down to recover and then you're released to go. More explaining and all questions answered. I like this part of the process

But then, just like that - SILENCE. It's like unplugging an instrument from an amp; that empty feedback sound. Yeah, that's about how it sounds in my head when I leave the clinic post transfer.

After being nurtured and communicated with daily, it comes to a screeching halt. Welcome to the hell of the TWW as an IVF patient. Going to the clinic, seeing your doctor and hearing updates on your body's progress, are part of your routine for weeks, or even months, leading up to the transfer. And then, just like that, you are dropped like a bad habit, for TWO WEEKS. I mean, it's outrageous; even though the clinic can't do anything more. It's a waiting game. What is one to do? I have gone through this FOUR TIMES, and the adjustment is a bitch every time. I find myself looking for things to fill my day. I think to myself, "I'm finally in the TWW, in the same position as a woman who is blessed to have babies the good-old fashioned way (which is all I have ever wanted), and now I HATE it."

I have realized over the last year that the IVF process has made me high maintenance when it comes to the TWW. I expect that same attention and frequent communication, and I am here to tell you, it isn't happening. I've had to learn to train my mind to slow down and be OK without daily updates. I have taken up meditation, written in my Five-Minute Journal, and practiced yoga. I have found ways to shift the focus to calming my body and mind to create a peaceful vessel for my embaby. For a girl who hates waiting and always needs answers, this is hard.

I know I'm not the only one out there like this. My advice to anyone following a similar path, is to find things you love to do that help slow down your mind and body. The gratitude and peace you can find while you wait will be gold. I will never be a girl who loves to wait, especially for two weeks, but I will do whatever it takes to get those two pink lines.

Blair Nelson @fabfertility

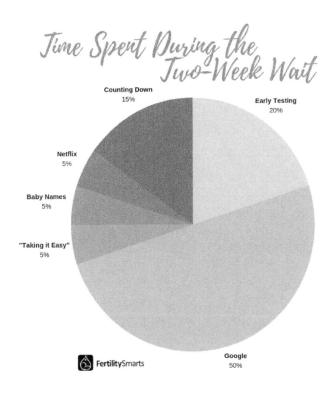

Time Spent During the Two-Week Wait

- Counting Down 15%
- Early Testing 20%
- Netflix 5%
- Baby Names 5%
- "Taking it Easy" 5%
- Google 50%

FertilitySmarts

Early tester or wait to test – Becky's view

So which camp do you sit in? Are you an eager early tester, or a patient 'official test-day' tester? According to a poll I recently carried out, 64% of my followers said they wait until test day. I have no idea how you do it!

My husband, Matt, and I sat in completely opposite camps – which was quite a challenge when the subject of discussion is possibly the most important test you will ever take together in your life. Obviously, emotion, (aka me!) overcame pragmatism, and we tested early, but we did spend a LOT of time debating the pros and cons of both options. You can read my (not so logical) emotionally driven account below, and Matt's view to wait, and wait, and wait, which is on the next page.

The TWW for me was never going to be two weeks. My reasons for testing early were three-fold and I'd recite these in my head, mainly to convince myself that I was doing the right thing! Writing about it now, I realise that my 'logic' seems pretty weak.

Firstly, I'd convinced myself that if I were to test early from the moment we returned home – and by early, I mean 9dp3dt (9 days post a 3-day transfer) or 6dp5dt, (6 days post a 5-day transfer) – I could still retain a glimmer of hope that the result might be a false negative. That way, I wouldn't experience the devastating blow of a definitive result on official test day (which someone once described to me as being like a 'sledge-hammer'). I almost preferred a trickle of negative results over a period of a few days, allowing the news to slowly sink in, rather than the sudden, terrifying fall from the mountain of built-up anticipation and hope.

Secondly, I've always believed that knowledge is power. If my embryo had implanted but hadn't developed, then I wanted to know, so I could feed this information back at the next 'WTF' clinic appointment. I wasn't sure whether anything could be done with this information, but I wanted to know as much as I possibly could about what was going on inside my body.

Thirdly, the prospect of knowing I was actually pregnant was far too tempting, being the impatient person that I am. I was simply too excited to wait to find out. You'd think the fear of the negative result would be greater, but for me, I don't believe it was. If I could have an answer that could end the pain, then I wanted it as soon as possible. That being said, after infertility, and experiencing a miscarriage, getting a positive test doesn't mean that suddenly the pain goes away, because you're now anxious that you ARE actually pregnant and it could still be snatched away.

So, there it is, I'd go with Matt's logical argument every time, but, as you all know, when it comes to IVF and TTC – rational thinking pretty much goes out of the window.

Becky Kearns @definingmum

Early tester or wait to test – Matt's view

Two weeks shouldn't be a huge deal in the greater scheme of things, but when your 'greater scheme' has been failure after failure for a few years, it can take on a whole new level of significance.

I'd consider myself a relatively level-headed pragmatist, so whilst Becky would happily have been testing twice-daily from the moment we got home, up to day fourteen, pleading with the stick to show a couple of lines, I was much more of the opinion that instead, we should wait out the duration, and then have a single 'moment of reveal'. On a practical level, this is what we'd been advised to do, and I certainly didn't want to test so early that the result would inevitably be negative, solely as things hadn't had time to develop to the extent that a positive result would even be possible.

The practical argument was predominantly employed as an excuse, however, as practicality very much takes a back seat once strong emotions exert their influence. A negative result would mean returning to the cycle that we'd become accustomed to with disappointment, soul-searching, grief and the dawning realisation that you're absolutely no nearer your goal…again.

For me, living in the glow of hope for a fortnight was infinitely preferable to experiencing the certainty of failure once more. Not knowing equated to not being disappointed for a brief period, and once you've been through a number of years of feeling frustrated and disillusioned, it was really nice just to experience some respite from this. Whilst Becky yearned for a moment of unbridled excitement, I was extremely content in dragging out the period of uncertainty as long as possible, as it removed the immediate need to put on a brave face and be 'the strong half' of the relationship, if things didn't go our way.

Matt Kearns

The two-week wait should be illegal

The two-week wait (TWW) is kind of like waiting for a call back from a job interview, except it happens once a month, and the answer is usually "No". Experiencing it once is painful enough, experiencing it over forty times should be illegal. I wouldn't wish it on anyone, and yet that's quickly becoming the norm for 1 in 8 couples struggling to conceive.

In my first two-week wait after fertility treatment, time stood still. I started doing pregnancy tests WAY too early, only to be disappointed every time I saw one line. I knew it was unreasonably soon, but I couldn't help it. I tried to busy myself with friends, date nights and writing, but nothing broke the baby spell I was under. I swear I felt something every time my stomach fluttered or popped or niggled. I was wrong. I wasn't pregnant. I was alone with my crazy hopes and obsessive imagination.

I read once that nature's cruellest trick is the similarities between pregnancy and PMS symptoms. I'm here to confirm that this couldn't be truer. My husband and I have been through too many TWW's to count, but the one thing I can count (on), is that it never gets easier.

Since the beginning of our trying to conceive, I have changed. I have lost myself in a way I would never have believed possible. And yet, in the same breath, I can confidently say that I've also become a much stronger version of me. Remember the phrase: 'If you get knocked down, you get up again'? That's what infertility and waiting is all about. Every month that 'it's a no', infertility knocks you back down. Every month that we proceed with an IUI, (intra uterine insemination), timed intercourse, an IVF cycle, (in vitro fertilisation), temperature tracking, peeing on ovulation sticks, and all the other paraphernalia, we choose to get back up again. Why? Because the reward is so much bigger than the journey we take to get there. The hope that someday 'soon' we'll have a baby in our arms, outweighs all the physical and emotional pain we endure to make our dream a reality.

Amelia Freeman @infertiltyblows

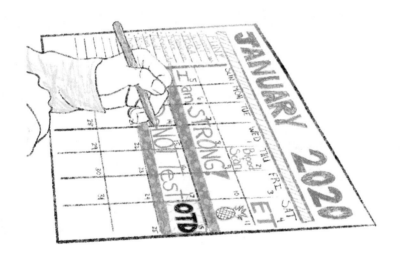

@sheilaalexanderart

31

A TWW post on an infertility forum

This post is fictional as are the usernames, any resemblance to actual usernames are purely coincidental.

HopefulICSI: TWW – and we're off again (*fingers crossed emoji*). Who's with me? I'm 3dp5dFET (soooo much quicker using abbreviations! *laughing emoji*). Hating the progesterone, feel sick & bloated. Popping them in the front entrance. Anyone tried the back entry? Wondering if better that way. Trying to enjoy being PUPO but so stressful when don't know what's going on in there. Has embaby stuck yet? Stick peanut, stick! Everyone else in the TWW, when are you testing? Good luck everyone.

RainbowMummy: I'm with you (*emoji with hand up*). 2dp3dt and I want to test already!! I know I can't and it's a waste of a hpt, but I need to feel like I'm doing something useful. I'll try and wait 'til 10dpt at least, though DH might have something to say about that! I did front last time so doing back entry as read that side effects not so bad. I hated the bloating, smelly farts (sorry TMI), sore boobs and sicky feeling – yeah pregnancy symptoms, so really hard to tell if it's worked this cycle. Wishing all a calm and beautiful TWW – is that even possible (*laughing emoji*).

HopefulICSI: Oh, maybe I'll ask my clinic if I can swap to back entry. Anything to make this time more bearable. Why oh why can't the 2WW pessaries make you feel positive and happy instead of bloated and nauseous? Have you got anything lovely planned to take you mind off it?

WaitingToConceive: Hi lovelies. I'm 4dp5dt and I tested out my trigger shot 2 days ago, so am testing every morning, first urine, and really hoping to see a faint line – please, please, please, (*fingers crossed emoji*). Crazy to do this I know, but I actually really loved testing as I got to see all those BFPs – might be the only time I do (*crying emoji*). I'm doing POI and am sooooo bloated, good job I'm lounging around in my pjs. Best of luck to us all (*prayer emoji*)

RainbowMummy: I'm taking some days off work HopefulICSI, having to take as holiday as work are not very supportive (*angry emoji*), so have lunch planned with a friend, who is in the know and very supportive (*thumbs up emoji and smiley emoji*). Going away for the weekend with OH and we have agreed no talking about IVF or pregnancy – that'll be hard! Then just going to watch some boxsets, read and cook nice healthy food (*heart emoji*). And you?

RainbowMummy: Oh, you're so brave WaitingToConceive! Last BFN cycle I didn't test at all, waited until beta, just wanted to stay in my happy-pretend-pregnant place and be in a bubble of PUPO (*kissing emoji*). This time I'm listening every day to an IVF relaxation app, really enjoying it and my DH says it's helping – not sure if he means me or him (*laughing emoji*).

Rachel456: Hi fellow wait-ers! I'm 2dp5dt, our 2nd fresh cycle. Sadly, we lost five embies between days 3 and 5 so nothing in the freezer as back up (*crying emoji*). I know for a fact that I'll be crazier by the end of this first week – my mind is constantly wondering what is happening, analysing every twinge, every different smell, an itchy nose, a bit of heartburn. I can't help but Dr Google it even though I know I shouldn't – no self-control me! Think for my marriage's sake I'll look into a relaxation app – thanks for the idea, RainbowMummy. Of course, I have my hpt's already to start testing, I'm too impatient to wait 'til OTD! Prayers and sticky embies to everyone (*heart emojis*)

HopefulICSI: Welcome to this exclusive club Rachel456!! Oh, so sorry to hear that you couldn't freeze any, so disappointing for you. Really up's the pressure doesn't it? I know what you mean about analysing, so hard not to! Anything different that I wasn't feeling an hour ago, I'm thinking must now be a sign. Right? I've been seeing a fertility coach, so I'm doing lots of visualisation – for 30 mins in the afternoon I have a lie down, place my hands on my tummy in a heart shape, visualise little peanut snuggling in, whisper all the things we're going to do together when they're born and how much I love him or her already. It's a really lovely thing to do and it's my time with my baby, (*lots of heart emojis*).

WaitingToConceive: I love that idea HopefulICSI (*heart emojis*),

I've not done visualisation before, sounds very relaxing, I'm definitely going to try it today. My head is all over the place, I can't concentrate, can't remember if I've already had some pineapple or not. Perhaps I should make a chart to help me remember *(laughing emojis)*.

Rachel456: *(Laughing emoji)* WaitingToConceive – another chart! Thank you HopefulICSI, yes, we were really optimistic that we would be able to freeze at least one, it's not much to ask is it? They all started so well, our hopes were high, then the phone call from the clinic to say they're weren't dividing any more *(crying emoji)*. Talk about a rollercoaster of emotions. Nothing can prepare you for the different levels you go through – from floating on clouds one minute to the depths of the ocean the next. Still it only takes one doesn't it? *(Fingers crossed emoji)*

Sheila @fertilitybooks

An excerpt from the book *The Pursuit of Motherhood*

The dreaded two-week wait: the period between your embryo transfer and pregnancy test, when time seems interminable. You become hyper-aware of every twinge, or lack of twinge, in your body, oscillating between thinking it's a good sign, then thinking it must be bad. Every physical movement or negative emotion feels like it might have jeopardised the process. You know that being positive is important, but you also don't trust yourself to deliver.

And then…

OUT DAMNED SPOT

For the first few days there's nothing.

You don't look.

You don't even think about looking.

Then, suddenly, a sign.

Faint at first.

Almost unnoticeable. Almost a surprise.

After that you start to look.

Dabbing for a few seconds longer than you need.

Peering intently.

In the beginning it's a light salmon pink.

Such a pretty, unoffending colour.

You google 'implantation bleeding'.

Persuade yourself that this is it.

A few hours pass. A day perhaps.

The pink continues.

Sometimes very visible. Sometimes less so.

And then something dark brown.

Small, solid, string-like.

You google 'implantation bleeding' again.

Persuade yourself that this is it.

Now you dab a little harder.

Really push around.

The pink is darker than it was, tinged with rust.

Then nothing.

No sign at all.

For a whole afternoon. A night, even.

Now you wipe more softly. Almost imperceptibly.

Just to prove that you're right.

That it's gone.

You start to feel positive.

You re-check the absence frequently.

Then leave it a little longer.

But then the salmon pink is back.

And suddenly, a streak of carmine red.

You google 'bleeding in early pregnancy'.

Read that it's relatively common.

Then another streak of red. And another.

Unavoidable. Undeniable.

You know nothing can survive it.

That the end of hope is near.

It doesn't matter how many times I'm told:

Stay positive. Everything may be OK.

I don't believe it.

I am Lady Macbeth. Guilty as charged.

Jessica Hepburn – author

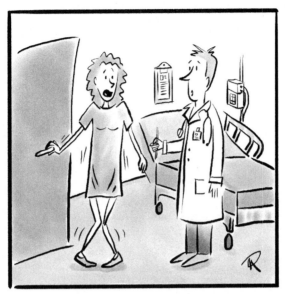

"Now, you absolutely promise
me it won't fall out?"

Top tips for the two-week wait (2WW)

'Should I work during my 2WW?' is the most common question
I'm asked, and my stock response is, 'There is no right or wrong
answer.'* I say this because I have worked, taken annual leave
and been unemployed through various 2WWs, all with the same
(negative) result. You need to make the decision of what's right
for you, and once you've done that, it's all about your mentality.

I went into my latest 2WW with one mantra; 'If this embryo
is going to stick, it's going to stick'. Because, let's face it, there
really is little we can do at this stage to make a difference.

Maybe it's because I've had my fair share of 2WWs over the
last six years that I've got to this stage, but the last one was
definitely the most successful - and I'm not talking in terms of

result, although admittedly, this has also been the best one so far too!

Yes, I've eaten pineapple core and guzzled down pomegranate juice, but the truth is, there's no real evidence I've seen that actually says these things will help. Don't get me wrong, I did feel like I was doing something positive which helped my mindset at the time, so, I'm not knocking it. The latest 2WW I guess, just put less pressure on what I was doing, and not doing, which helped my mindset in a completely different way.

Even with this attitude, it isn't easy. I don't know about you, but for me, following the relative 'breeze' of week one, when week two rolls around, it's definitely more difficult. The lead up to test day is intense and, unlike some I know, I'm not a tester, so it all comes down to that last day, or OTD as its commonly called in the community.

Here are my top tips for that second week in particular:

- Distraction is the name of the game: plan activities, visit friends, play board games, eat out, whatever works for you, distract yourself!

- 'No Regrets' - my mantra throughout our years of treatment. If something doesn't feel right - or does – follow your gut instinct. It doesn't matter what anyone else tells you, (unless it's backed up by rigorously tested research of course, then you probably should listen). But research aside, there are so many dos and don'ts; some will feel right, some won't, and at the end of the day, it's you who needs to live with your decisions.

- Don't test early. I know lots of people do, but I just wonder why you would put yourself through the anguish, over several days, when you know the test is measuring the hormone hCG (human chorionic gonadotrophin) level, which isn't reliable before the two weeks are up.

- One thing I do know; whatever the result, you are not alone, and you will get through the next few weeks and months, even if it may not feel like it at the time.

*Caveat to this statement, is that if you work in a physical job, I would at the very least, reduce some of the physicality.

Cat Strawbridge @tryingyears

Now let's play a fun 2WW game - Hunt the symptom!

Contestant: Amber, aged 34, IVF, 1st cycle

Implantation bleeding? – What does implantation bleeding even look like? Is it like spotting, or like a period? Is it dark, bright or watery blood? The resulting Google image search was a clear reminder that it isn't possible to un-see things. Up popped photos of people's gungy, bloodied tissues. Gross, don't Google it. But I needed to compare other people's implantation bleeding to … to what? I didn't have any. So why was I Googling it?

Cramps? – The departure from the norm were cramps around twelve hours after egg transfer, which I put down to my womb making a justified objection to having a stick wiggled around inside it earlier in the day. Fair play. A few twinges here and there, but it could have just been tight pants. I had squeezed my bloated hippo arse into a new set of knickers, necessitated by ruining all my old comfy ones with progesterone pessaries. An embryo implanting or a tight bit of elastic? It was anyone's guess.

Constant weeing? – I was plagued by the need for night-time wees. This can sometimes be a symptom of early pregnancy, and so whilst my newly acquired (and very annoying) nocturnal habit should have brought some comfort, it didn't. The reason being that the explanation for frequent urination in early pregnancy is likely to be hormonal, caused by the presence of hCG (human Chorionic Gonadotrophin hormone) and increased progesterone. What IVF does is artificially pump hCG into your system via the trigger shot, and a high dose of regularly self-administered progesterone. Add to that the need to stay hydrated by drinking approximately two litres of water per day, and I'm sorry pee … but I just couldn't trust what you were telling me. IVF is in itself wee inducing.

Increased heart rate? – Not properly measured, but I felt like my heart rate was up, sometimes a possible indication of early pregnancy. It is also an indication of an extremely stressed lady suffering through a never-ending two-week wait.

Feeling like your period is coming? – This was what clinched it for me. My expectations of a successful result plummeted as that all too familiar feeling crept into my uterus. I could feel my period coming. For me it's a heavy, full, churning feeling, like a storm brewing in my womb. This sensation usually arrives around five to seven days prior to the arrival of Aunt Flo, and like clockwork it started up a week into my two-week wait. In my mind that was it! I knew that early pregnancy can feel like your period, that progesterone could mirror pregnancy symptom's, and anything can mean everything, or nothing at this stage. You just can't tell, because it all feels the same.

Amber Woodward, @thepreggerskitchen

Why we feel the way we do during the two-week wait

The two-week wait or 2WW is one of the most challenging times in a fertility journey. It's that time after your egg has been fertilised, and you have to wait to find out if the embryo has implanted in your uterus, or not. The 2WW occurs after fertility treatment (IVF – in vitro fertilisation, IUI – intra uterine insemination), when an embryo has been transferred, or when you're trying to get pregnant naturally, and you have timed intercourse with ovulation. It's a time of hope, anxiety, uncertainty, and stress. You may also feel extra attentive to body signs — like pain, aches, spotting, tenderness — and feel the need to interpret them as signs of early pregnancy, or lack of. The reality is that we can't attribute these signs to the presence or not of a pregnancy. A number of women who have these physical signs see a positive pregnancy test at the end of the two weeks, but others experiencing the same symptoms get a negative pregnancy test. The same can be said if you don't feel any symptoms. You may get a positive or a negative pregnancy test.

Taking a home pregnancy test before the two weeks are up is not advisable, because these tests detect hCG (human Chorionic Gonadotrophin hormone) in your urine, which is a hormone produced when the embryo implants in your womb. This hormone is also present in some fertility medications, so if you test early, you may see a positive pregnancy test even though you are not pregnant; or you may have a negative test when you are actually pregnant, but the levels of the hormone are still too low to be detected by the home test.

So, if you can't gain comfort in early signs or early pregnancy tests, what can you do to cope with the emotions triggered during this time? The first step is understanding why we feel the way we do. Psychology explains this with the memories, values and beliefs we hold, which make us see the world a certain way. The way we see the world triggers certain feelings, which make us take certain actions, and get certain results.

When you are going through the two-week wait, you know you have been trying for a baby for a while and are hoping for a positive result. However, the challenges you've been through so far have also affected your beliefs around this experience, so even though you may feel hopeful, you may also feel anxious, or feel that it's not going to work. These feelings will make you take certain actions (conscious or unconscious), which may affect the results at the end of the two-week wait.

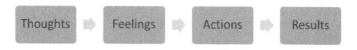

Thoughts ➡ Feelings ➡ Actions ➡ Results

Acknowledging the beliefs and thoughts that aren't helpful to you is the first step to having a calmer and more peaceful two-week wait. Write down the thoughts that are making you feel anxious, stressed, sad or any other unhelpful emotion, alongside the intensity of the emotion from 1 to 10. The next step is to write down the evidence that supports that thought and feeling. We do this naturally, so it won't be difficult to find why you're thinking the way you are. Then, look for evidence that negates that thought: it may be that this time you've done things differently, prepared your body or that the embryo was a better grade. Finally, notice how the initial emotion has changed. This exercise is the first step to taking control of that tiny voice in your head, and then changing it to be more supportive of what you are going through.

Thought	Emotion (/10)	Evidence that supports my thought	Evidence that refutes my thought	Conclusion	Emotion (/10)
This embryo transfer is not going to work	Hopelessness (10/10) Sadness (10/10)	My previous embryo transfer didn't work and I'm feeling the same way	I did a lot of different things in preparation for this embryo transfer. This embryo was a better quality. My friend had the same symptoms and had a positive test.	Even though I don't have any new symptoms, I have done a lot of different things preparing my body for this transfer, and the embryo was good quality	Hopelessness (5/10) Sadness (5/10)

Andreia Trigo @infertile_life

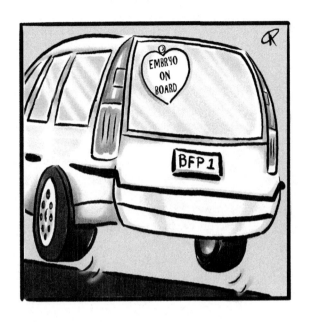

Journaling through the two-week wait

The two-week wait (2WW) is super tough. What really got me through mine was my journal. I had never been particularly enthusiastic about journaling, but during my IVF (in-vitro fertilisation) cycles, it literally kept me (almost) sane.

First of all, I made a page of my journal into a 2WW advent calendar, so I could cross off each day that took me nearer to test day.

I also used my journal as a place to offload all my anxiety. It was really therapeutic as a space where I could just let rip and 'get it all out'. I always felt better after that. Sometimes I processed events that had happened; or I wrote down what I would really have liked to say to the person who had wound me up that day – usually by telling me to 'just relax'. My journal was about naming my hopes and dreams, and witnessing them for myself.

I also copied affirmations and words of encouragement into my journal when I came across particularly good ones. Just the process of writing them down was useful, but it also meant that I knew I had them to hand when I needed them. Affirmations such as: 'Just for today, I will not worry', and belief statements such as: 'I am fertile and strong,' were a really useful focus for my overactive mind.

My journal was also a creative space where I activated my imagination. My training as a creative therapist had shown me just how powerful it can be to access the subconscious mind through creative practice, and I wanted to harness that magic. I have some wild pictures from that time! There's a cartoon drawing of my two embryos implanting themselves into my womb and calling out, "Hello Mum," and another self-portrait, where I am sending love to my womb. I'm no artist by any stretch of the imagination, but the process of drawing was relaxing in its own way, and I believe that it helped me to engage my whole self in the positive visualisation of a successful pregnancy.

The two-week wait is always going to be difficult, but there are ways that you can support yourself. Listen to your own intuition as to what will be most beneficial for you. If you decide to journal, there is no right or wrong way to go about it. You can write in an exercise book, use a sketchpad or treat yourself to one of the many fabulous specialist IVF diaries and journals on the market, which provide helpful prompts and templates.

Sending you all love and luck

Emma xx

Dr Emma Brodzinski @dremmabrodzinski

Me and my two-week waits

Patience has never been my strong point. In fact, I would go as far as to say I have no patience at all. So, each time I have found myself in the TWW, both naturally and through treatment, I have always tested early. I never used to wait for my period to arrive when we were trying naturally, and I have never waited until 'Official Test Day' during treatment.

I don't beat myself up about that either. I've accepted that I would rather know as soon as possible than wait. The problem with testing so early is that you can create extra anxiety. You can have a false negative, and I have spent far too much money on pregnancy tests hoping to see a strong line show up. But each time, I don't listen to that rational side of my brain, I continue to test early. If that's your personality too, then don't worry, you are not alone.

Distraction has always helped me keep relatively calm within the TWW. I plan nice things and make sure I don't spend too much time not doing much. Mentally I need to keep busy, as the moment I'm left alone with my thoughts, the negativity creeps in. I've seen some people write plans, so they have many wonderful daily activities, which I think is a great thing to do. After embryo transfers, I like to rest for twenty-four hours, then resume normal life, albeit at a gentle pace. Side effects from the drugs can leave you feeling quite groggy, so it can be hard to muster up some energy, but it has always been important for me to try and keep active.

During the TWW for my first IVF cycle, I went back to work during the second week, and it was a wonderful distraction. At the time I had a desk job, so no major physical activity, and it was lovely to be busy. Although it's important to fuel your body with healthy and nutritious food and drink, I think it's also important not to beat yourself up if you fancy a treat. There is always so much guilt surrounding diet with trying to conceive, and I think the key is moderation. To deprive yourself of what you love can add more stress to your metal health, so it's important to remember to be kind to yourself.

It can feel like the longest two weeks ever, so it's important to take it day by day. Try not to focus on that end date too much and most importantly, remember to live!

Kate @mrskmeaks

To test or not to test? That is the question

We have all struggled with the awful two-week wait, and the question of whether to test or not. This urge to pee-on-a-stick usually pops up around 7 or 8 DPO, (days post ovulation), and even though we know that the possibility of a pregnancy being detected at this point is essentially zero, we still do it. We waste our money and quite frankly, compromise our sanity. Then we don't believe the negative result anyway. All we prove to ourselves is that, yes, it was too early to test and we will re-test in a couple of days.

By the time we get to 12DPO, we start to believe the negative test a little bit more, (though still not fully), but part of the continued testing at this stage is to manage our expectations. If I am prepared for the negative, it will hurt less when my period arrives. At least this part is a little bit true.

Then add Google into the mix. Am I the only one who has found themselves in some weird Google chat room reading about people who didn't get a positive test until they were eight weeks pregnant? Or reading up on people who got their period, but were still pregnant after all? Maybe I am one of these people. Maybe the test just won't register that I am pregnant. Yeah, that must be it.

I can say this, because I have lived it.... peeing-on-sticks is insanity. We pull our hair out deciding whether or not to test, followed by testing, and then not believing the result.

Our misery ends when Aunt Flo (period) arrives, and then sometimes, we even question THAT.

I made a promise to myself about six months ago: no more testing. It adds nothing to my life, and actually, takes a lot away. I truly wish I had learned this earlier in my TTC journey. It is everyone's choice to test or not to test, and you have to choose what's right for you. I just challenge you to think about whether it's adding to your life or taking away from it. And if it's the latter, then put your emotional well-being at the top of your priority list and toss those tests into the trash.

@HerFertilityDiary

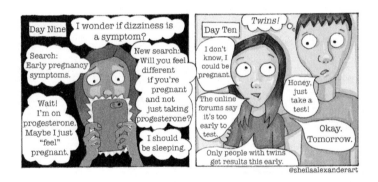

The two-week wait is stressful

The 2-week wait is horrendous; probably the main reason I don't want to do any more fertility treatments. It's too stressful and puts so much pressure on both of us. Every day we were worried about what my wife was doing, what she was eating, making sure she didn't do too much. Any twinge was a massive deal. There was nothing we could do to take our minds off it. We are desperate to have children and infertility has completely taken over our lives for the last three to four years.

The blighted ovum was horrific. With the first one, my wife had every pregnancy symptom. Blood and urine tests confirmed she was pregnant, so we went to our 7-week viability scan expecting to see an embryo. Because we'd had two embryos transferred, I was thinking I'd be disappointed if there was only one; I was hoping for two. To then be told there was an empty sac… we were devastated. We thought because she had all the symptoms and the tests said she was pregnant, we believed there was a baby. No one told us that this may not be the case.

The second blighted ovum, we believed again she was pregnant. Apparently, a blighted ovum is quite rare, so we didn't think we could be that unlucky. Finding out this news on our last attempt on the NHS was again devastating. I felt like I'd been kicked in the stomach. Nearly six months later, it's still upsetting to talk about. I know losing a baby much later can be worse, and people think at seven weeks a miscarriage can't be that painful, but believe me, it is. And IVF (in-vitro fertilisation) makes it ten times worse.

Gareth James, UK

EXTRACT FROM THE BLOG: 'Seven Infertility Helpers from Hell'

If you are going through a two-week wait after fertility treatment, you've probably been dealing with infertility prior to this point, so I'm absolutely certain that you've come across at least one, if not more, infertility helpers from hell. These 'helpers' don't let up even when you're in a two-week wait. If you know someone who's struggled with infertility and waiting to find out if they are pregnant, then you may, or may not, recognise yourself as an infertility helper from hell. Sorry, I don't mean to offend. An infertility helper from hell is a person who means well, but who hinders your healing. Their intentions may be good, but their efforts often turn out to be self-absorbed and, ultimately, unhelpful. Here I respectfully offer, 'Seven Infertility Helpers from Hell'.

1. **The Fixer**—The Fixer is certain that your terrible situation is a question and they know the answer. In fact, this person has ALL the answers to how to heal from your predicament. Note that I called this a predicament, not your fear and pain. For them, this is a project to be figured out. There's a blueprint. Just do what they recommend, be grateful, and you will be A-OK. Doesn't that make you feel all warm and fuzzy from your head to your toes? And you better feel good, real quick. I remember when The Fixer told my husband and me to make love on the beach under a full moon and we'd get pregnant. I couldn't make this up. The answer has been offered. What are you waiting for? Get to it. And Don't-Worry-About-It! Unfortunately, your spouse may be a Fixer. The Fixer needs you to take their advice and feel good, because he or she is already thinking about their own life, and it's too difficult to even imagine what you're going through. They can't. They'd rather work on you as a goodwill project than consider the possibility of fear and pain in their own lives.

2. **The Comparer**—The Comparer knows a person with PCOS who GOT PREGNANT on their FIRST IVF cycle and then they GOT PREGNANT again ON THEIR OWN and they KNOW that you will too! They don't know how they know this, but they sure do. Because the Comparer refuses to accept that your predicament is personal—and yes, (ahem) many vaginal ultrasounds and semen samples are personal — this person needs to deflect your personal pain. It would be really painful for this person to feel your pain. This person will not win a gold medal in validation or empathy. They file you into a category for which they have a reference. They may also talk about how they are the same as you, because something really bad happened to them in their life, like whiplash, or they didn't get that job they really wanted. And they were very, very sad. FYI, your pain is about them, too. The Comparer can't deal with the intense feelings that you are dealing with, and it's easier to talk about themselves or someone else who also has a really, really, really hard story. Even harder than your own, of course.

3. **The Reporter**—The Reporter wants all the juicy details. "Oooooh, tell me more?" they say. They have many questions, ranging from the curious to the spicy, and they await your detailed answers. This is a Pulitzer prize winning New York Times reporter with a spiral notebook and a digital recorder. And once The Reporter has the data, they just CANNOT keep a secret. They have to share your big, horrible story with others without your consent. "Did you hear? Isn't that JUST AWFUL?" The Reporter shares with boundaryless abandon in the spirit of transparency, because she or he is just so darn worried about you. Really, it's easier to tell a story than to feel your pain.

4. **The Cricket**—*sound of crickets*. I am whispering. This person is quiet because they don't know what to do, or say, or ask. They don't want to do anything that might make you feel worse. So, they do nothing. But they may say they heard you were doing okay, from The Reporter maybe? And they

are hoping against hope that that's true, because they don't know what to do, or say, or ask.

5. **God Reps**—Everybody take a breath and please don't curse me out. I'm just a messenger here. The God Rep is on a gossamer trail of thoughts and prayers, straight from The Big One upstairs. This person knows how you should feel. Isn't that a relief? God knows why you are in this predicament, according to the God Rep. They feel called upon by the Lord to tell you that God has a plan for you. The suffering of trying to conceive for years and spending a bucket of money on having children is part of the plan. Isn't it that simple? I have seen many good people, devout people, get violently furious about the God Rep's very important message. Did you know that you can have a conversation with God directly, without the God Rep's 'help', and that you can feel, however you feel, good or bad? The Big One can handle all of your feelings.

6. **The Cheerleader**—Yay! You are going to be okay! They just know it! Turn that frown upside down! Rah! You have time! You are young! You are going to beat the odds! This is gonna work! You just gotta think positive! You just need to put on your lipstick and 'relax and eat your vegetables and do acupuncture!'. The Cheerleader is too uncomfortable to step out of their rosy formation to consider your reality. They don't understand that they are dismissing your every emotion and leaving you feeling quite alone.

7. **The Victim**—The Victim has heard about your terrible news and feels just awful — wait for it — that you didn't share your news directly with them. They had to hear second-hand. They are overcome with emotion. They are so distraught about being left out of your big story that they need to breathe for a moment. They thought you were close. They need to tell you how they feel. Please note that they haven't expressed any empathy for YOUR frustration and grief. Theirs is bigger. Much bigger.

Who is the real helper when you feel vulnerable and afraid?

It's the person who just listens, who gives you a hug without offering advice. The Real Helper goes to the clinic with you, just because. They cry with you, because infertility is unfair, and they know you hurt. It's the person who offers understanding, not judgment. They ask and understand when you can't talk about it today. They hold out hope for you, and your future when you feel hopeless. They don't offer to give you one of their children. They give what they can give in the hope that it's helpful to you somehow, maybe now, maybe later. And this person keeps checking in, offering a smile or an open ear.

Sometimes you have to be very clear with people about what you need. Like me, East Coast Debbie. In the words of the immortal Spice Girls, "I'll tell you what I want, what I really, really want." What most people are desperate for is EMPATHY. The Real Helpers do exist. Please take the risk and open your heart to them.

Dr Deborah Simmons @partners_in_fertility

Seven tips to surviving the 2WW

Based on my own IVF (in-vitro fertilisation) journey of five cycles, I learned that stress is one of the biggest and most difficult issues to handle. By being aware of knowing that you can't control the waiting time, the best thing to do is make space to create and find opportunities.

Here are seven tips to survive your 2WW and make it an easier one:

1. Go easy after your transfer – start journaling, and if you already do, make it better by writing your own story. Journaling and writing how we are feeling every step of our journey, helps us immensely, to release not only the emotional distress and anxiety of the cycle, but also leaves

space in our mind and heart to be able to create and fill it with more positive thoughts and manifestations.

2. Eat well, rest, but also remember that you are not sick, so take a nice walk along the beach, in the woods or just down the street. It's proven that exercise and appreciation of nature elevate the levels of serotonin (our happy hormone), in our brain, which helps us to open our minds and allow colorful thoughts in. Your mind remembers beautiful images, so when you go for a walk along the beach or in nature, what you see stays in your brain, like an image in a camera. This creates positivity and reduces stress.

3. Please do not test early as this puts more pressure and stress on yourself. Wait until your beta test. I know this is a difficult one, I have been there, but the best way I managed to hold out was to create challenges for myself when I was tempted to test. So, every time I had the urge to run to the pharmacy and buy a pregnancy test, I would focus on something I enjoyed. For me, this was coloring or beading. I love to make beads and stone bracelets.

4. Color and create: art therapy is an excellent tool to release stress and focus our mind on something positive. Just as I mentioned above, opening our minds to creativity increases our serotonin and distracts our mind from negative and stressful thoughts. Trust me, even if you aren't an 'artistic individual' you have some creative gift in your heart — look for it, feel it — even by doing this, you're already occupying your mind with something that can take you away from the stress of this journey.

5. Watch comedy movies with your partner; this makes time go faster and you'll also be enjoying yourself. Laughing is conceivable, (that's even the title of a book from my good friend, Lori Shandle-Fox, and is about how she made IVF a fun and humorous journey). But my point here is that we MUST allow ourselves to smile and laugh during this time, because the more we do this, the more we're increasing our chances to make this pregnancy a successful one.

Remember, technically you're pregnant once your embryo is transferred, so think that way. If you laugh, then your embaby laughs too as you create a nice warm and happy womb for it.

6. Pamper yourself, have a foot massage*, a pedicure, a manicure, your makeup done, feel the beauty you have that's inside you. This is about being kind and taking care of yourself. Why? Because if we don't, it's like we're not preparing the home for our rainbow baby. If we look sad, or feel ugly, or just crap, that's the home we are preparing for our baby. So, if you take care of yourself, and pamper yourself, you are doing the same for the embaby that's inside your beautiful womb.

7. Acupuncture* is a great option too, along with meditation or chill-out music, and a beautiful tool for peace and ease. I did many sessions of this incredible technique on my last IVF cycle, and I truly think it was a big part of why I was successful. This helps you to quieten your mind and train your brain to be in the moment. The more you do it, the better you become at relaxing. Try it weekly from the beginning of your treatment, and then twice a week during your 2WW. When quietening your mind, you are in a state of peace and tranquillity.

* Always check with your health practitioner prior to having any other treatments.

Monica Bivas @monicabivas

After a 5-day transfer, what is that embryo doing?

During an IVF (in-vitro fertilisation) cycle, eggs are collected from your ovaries and are fertilised by the sperm in some manner. Once fertilised, which occurs within the first eighteen hours, your clinic calls you to tell you how many have fertilised. This is a nerve-wracking call. The fertilised eggs are regularly checked by the embryologist, and a decision will be made as to when you have your transfer. Transfer usually take place on Day 2, Day 5 or sometimes Day 6.

Day 1 (transfer day): Officially the embryo is called a 'blastocyst' but 'blasty' doesn't sound as cute! So, we'll stick with embaby, who is busy beginning to hatch out of his or her shell, somewhere in your womb. You are PUPO (pregnant until proven otherwise). Yay!

Day 2: Embaby is still busy and spends the day hatching out of his or her shell, and, a big development happens as he or she also begins to attach to your womb; exact position unknown. You're in love already. But don't test yet.

Day 3: Embaby is working hard and attaches deeper to your womb lining – this means implantation is beginning. Exciting! But don't test yet.

Day 4: Embaby continues to implant somewhere in your womb. Love. Love. Love. And don't test yet – there's a reason why I keep saying this.

Day 5: At last, implantation is complete. Embaby has also been busy developing cells that will become the placenta, and some more cells that will become your baby – at just five days old! What a busy bee. But don't test yet.

Day 6: Human chorionic gonadotrophin, or hCG for short, (thank goodness for abbreviations), is known as the pregnancy hormone, which now starts to enter your bloodstream. That's why I kept saying: 'Don't test yet', because your embaby hasn't started making their own hCG yet.

Day 7: Your baby continues to develop and more hCG enters your bloodstream. Yay! You CAN test soon.

Day 8: Your baby continues to develop and more hCG enters your bloodstream. Yay – again!

Day 9: The levels of hCG are now high enough in your bloodstream for a blood test to show a BFP. YOU CAN TEST NOW! Good luck.

Sheila@fertilitybooks

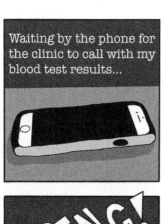

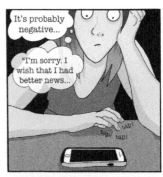

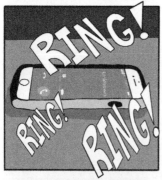

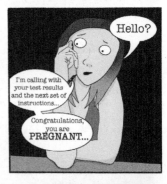

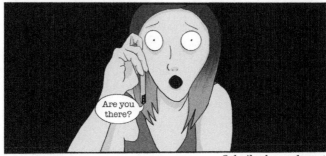

The TWW for women with irregular cycles

Having irregular cycles adds an extra layer of complexity to getting pregnant, and it can mean that you have no idea when your TWW is, or you feel even more pressure during your TWW, as they happen less often.

Getting to know your cycle

With irregular cycles, it can be helpful to track them using the Basal Body Temperature method to confirm ovulation. Using Ovulation Predictor Kits (OPK) can be a very expensive and an often ineffective way of predicting ovulation. It's really helpful to understand that it's the first part of your cycle, (the follicular phase - first day of your period up to ovulation), that is the irregular part, and that the second part of your cycle, (the luteal phase - ovulation to period) i.e. the TWW, is pretty consistent.

Once you understand when/if your body ovulates, you will be able to recognise your body's cues around ovulation, which will help you time your sexual activity. Some cues to look for are small pains/cramps on the left or right side of your abdomen, egg white cervical mucus and increased libido. Learn what your ovulation signs are.

The added pressure

If you are able to work out when your TWW is, it can feel like your whole world is on hold because it happens less frequently for you. You can feel like you have to 'do everything right' when it does come around. It's understandable that you feel pressure, but it's OK to live your life too. You don't need to put everything on hold. You don't need to do everything perfectly.

The most important thing you can do during this time is to be kind to yourself. Each day check in with yourself and see what you need. This could be as basic as having a drink of water or asking those around you for support to get your emotional needs met.

Sometimes it can be helpful to switch your focus during this time. Is there an old hobby that you'd like to try again? Any crafting projects that you'd love to spend a bit more time on? Are there some friends you'd love to catch up with? Find the things that fill you with joy and energy and prioritise doing these things. And if all you feel like doing is staying at home and watching Netflix - find an epic comedy that makes you laugh out loud.

The not knowing

If you are unsure if you ovulate and if you even have a TWW, it's completely normal to feel resentful of others for even getting that far. It's OK to acknowledge and accept this feeling. It doesn't make you a bad person. It can feel frustrating that you have no idea what is going on with your body. If you are able to, ensure that you are getting support from your doctor about your ovulation.

Something that can be helpful during this time is to find other ways to get in touch with your body. Some ways you can start to tune into your body are:

- Practicing yoga: even a few simples stretches can bring more awareness to your body

- Meditating: you can get guided meditation apps like Calm or Headspace, or just take a moment, close your eyes and take four big deep breaths

- Tracking your mood: Tracking how you feel on a daily basis can help you to notice what things in your life affect your mood, and what small adjustments you can make every day to improve your mood and wellbeing.

Finding others that are experiencing the same frustrations as you, can be really helpful to support you through the particular challenges that come with having irregular cycles.

Nicola Salmon @fatpositivefertility

Prioritise your emotional wellbeing

Like many people, I found that infertility changed my outlook on life, and forced me to reassess my goals and the areas in which I wanted to invest my time and energy. This is one of the few benefits of infertility, (although it certainly doesn't feel as though there are any benefits at the time). It encouraged me to stop sleepwalking through life, stop making assumptions and taking things for granted, and start to experience greater clarity in terms of what mattered, what didn't, and who I wanted to be as a person.

Why is it so hard?

I think everyone can understand the physical toll that IVF takes: the injections, the influx of hormones, the uncomfortable procedures, and the driving to and from appointments. The impact on your relationship if you're part of a couple is also easily recognised; the stress of trying to get pregnant; the fear of fertility investigations and their results; the blame that can be attributed to one or both parties, and the financial strain. But what I've learned is that there are subtle strands in the tangle of emotions we experience that are rarely, if ever, described when we sign up to IVF, and it's important to recognise them if we're going to support ourselves effectively.

IVF forces us to put our hearts on the line

Normally, when people decide to try for a baby, it's something personal and private, a monumental decision kept closely under wraps.

But in an IVF cycle, the situation is very different. We are forced to declare to ourselves, all the staff at our fertility clinic, and often family, friends and work colleagues, that there is one thing we want more than anything else – a baby! And that we are willing to invest in it, physically, emotionally, and sometimes financially, even though the odds of success are not in our favour. This is a pretty unnatural way to manage our greatest hopes and aspirations, which we would much prefer to protect and keep close to our hearts, at least until we feel that we have some control over making them happen.

With our natural defences stripped away, we face the two-week wait with an intense feeling of vulnerability and powerlessness, and a growing fear of failure if it doesn't work out.

These feelings are some of the most uncomfortable for human beings to endure, so if you find yourself feeling anxious, argumentative or just generally fragile in the two-week wait, then you should know that you're experiencing a very normal human response to the situation you find yourself in.

It's isolating

The two-week wait in particular, is an isolating time. If you spend the time at home, you may feel physically isolated, and even if you're surrounded by colleagues at work, many people report that they feel very much alone. Similarly, if you tell your friends and family about your treatment, there's often a limit to how much of your experience they'll be able to understand. For anyone going through IVF without a partner, the isolation can be particularly pronounced, since there is nobody else invested in the outcome to the extent that you are.

Sympathy is stifling

While we all value genuine support, there's nothing worse than unwanted pity. One of the top concerns that seems to prevent people from seeking support from others is that they don't want people to feel sorry for them. Many people lack trust in their manager or HR department, and the thought of becoming the subject of office gossip or pitying glances from across a meeting room forces them to invent excuses for taking time off work and attempting to carry on as though nothing significant is happening. This is a heavy burden to carry because, when you're in the two-week wait, it's hard to deny that something very significant is happening in your life.

It can be hard to support somebody else when you're struggling yourself

Going through IVF with a partner can be a wonderful source of support, or an additional strain, or sometimes a combination of both. Many people feel they must 'be strong' for their partner and suppress their own fears and concerns, whilst others find that arguments are easily triggered during the two-week wait – not surprising when there is so much stress and anxiety beneath the surface for both partners.

This is another reason why being forewarned is being forearmed; knowing what to expect, and why arguments are likely to come about can help both of you to accept and withstand any rough patches you might go through.

How to prioritise your emotional wellbeing

Having support in place from the outset is always going to feel easier than trying to reach out for it when you're already feeling overwhelmed. Ahead of your two-week wait, it can be worthwhile to map out a support network around you, ensuring, if possible, that there's someone you can turn to in all the important areas of your life:

- **Work life**

  If you're planning to work through the two-week wait, it may help to speak to your manager ahead of time, to explain that you won't know how you'll feel, and may need to take time off with short notice, avoid physically strenuous work, or take more of a back seat in projects and meetings where possible. If you have a 'Plan B' from the beginning, you're less likely to feel guilty or trapped into continuing a heavy workload when deep down you know you need a break.

  If you have a particularly stressful job or a manager you feel unable to talk to, you may find it helpful to speak to your GP about getting signed off for the duration of the two-week wait. Fertility Network UK has launched an initiative called Fertility in the Workplace, helping you to speak to your HR department if there is no existing policy in place to support you through fertility treatment. See their website for more information www.fertilitynetworkuk.org

- **Home Life**

   If you have a partner it can be helpful to plan some time together – time that doesn't involve fertility appointments, injections or other reminders of treatment. If your relationship is feeling the strain – which is very common – couples counselling may be a valuable source of support and help you to reconnect and to understand how you both truly feel about what's happening. You don't necessarily have to attend the sessions together either; you can attend individual sessions, joint sessions, or a mixture of the two. What's important is that you can talk to each other, and also both have someone else to lean on when you need an outside perspective, or some extra support.

   If you don't have a partner, it's important to identify early on who your 'rock' or 'rocks' are going to be – people close to you who will know what you're going through and will be available to provide comfort, reassurance or just good company when you need it.

- **Social Life**

   Identify the people and things in your life that lift you up, make you laugh and generally make you forget your worries, if only for a while. Remind yourself that, as part of your IVF support network, these are the people that it's worth reaching out to, even if you feel that you don't want to leave the house for two weeks.

- **Spiritual Life**

   You don't need to belong to a particular faith to connect with your spirituality, and it's something that naturally comes to the fore during the two-week wait, as we are focused on trying to create a new life, and therefore on the meaning and purpose of our own lives.

It's good to identify what your 'soul food' might be, whether it's a walk by the sea or in nature, taking time to meditate or pray, curling up under a blanket with a favourite book or film, or drawing strength from all the memories of the people throughout your life whom you've loved, and who've loved you … and given you inspiration.

Rachel Cathan @rachelcathancounselling, Author of *336 Hours*

Surviving the two-week wait (2WW)

I think there are two main categories people fall into regarding the 2WW. The first are those who want to test, test, test every day in the hope of getting a positive pregnancy result, and there are those who would rather live in ignorant bliss, and have an aversion to testing. I fall into the second category, and I'm not sure if it's because I have had both positive and negative tests and know the feeling of utter desolation on getting a BFN, (big fat negative). Or, if it's because I've had three miscarriages and an ectopic pregnancy, and I'm actually scared of both results.

As I do fall into the 'no news is good news' category, I'm usually OK with the 2WW. I don't mind the not knowing if I'm pregnant or not, especially as test day looms; but there is no denying that for everyone it's a difficult two-week period. One of the main reasons the 2WW is so hard is due to the medications – namely progesterone – that brings about pregnancy-type symptoms, such as tiredness, sore boobs, twinges and mild nausea. You start to believe you are pregnant, which makes a BFN a bitter pill to swallow.

So, what can you do to survive?

- Diet and nutrition: focusing on diet not only helps pass the time, but has a really positive impact on mental health. By growing and buying the best quality products (preferably organic) you can afford, you know you are doing everything you can to ensure your embaby or embabies have the best possible chance. During the 2WW, I enjoyed baking my favourite healthy recipes, finding new recipes to try out in pregnancy and TTC books, and developing new smoothies, juices and salads – pineapple cores are meant to be amazing post-transfer as they contain the enzyme bromelain which may help embryos stick. If you have a nutritionist, and even better, if she or he is a specialist in fertility, they will be able to suggest recipes to help. Don't beat yourself up if you fancy a treat – these two weeks are all about nurture, comfort and nourishment, and this goes for your soul too. If you want a chocolate brownie, have a chocolate brownie! It's all about balance and not deprivation.

- Supplements: It's really important to adjust your supplements during this time – I see this as setting yourself up for success and helping embryo development. Spend your time doing some research, seek advice from a qualified nutritionist and talk to friends in the TCC community – it is the most supportive community.

- Destress your environment: Reducing stress is really important throughout the whole process of IVF and no more so than in the 2WW. I made the decision not to work through each of my 2WW's, as I didn't want work stress to impact my outcome. Some people find working through really helpful, as it helps distract them, but if, like me, you are prone to stress and letting outside factors get to you, try to avoid them if possible and manage your environment, e.g. work from home if you can.

A friend of mine finds taking a holiday helps – nothing is more distracting than a new environment, and who doesn't love a holiday? It can really help you relax. The best advice I can give, as an old pro, is to avoid people and situations which cause you stress, especially if someone is negative or not supportive – just don't do it. Avoid, at all costs, social occasions which could possibly upset you –

you are number one in this process so don't feel obligated to do ANYTHING, other than look after yourself, your embryo(s) and your mental health.

- Arts and crafts: To some this may sound twee, but creating something is incredibly rewarding. Painting, drawing, sketching, knitting, chalk painting, sewing and the like are very gentle nurturing ways to pass the 2WW – after all, creating something new is exactly what your body is doing. Using your creative skills, whether good or bad, it's not a competition, so who cares how your endeavours turn out; it's the 'doing' that's important, so just relax and have fun.

- Gentle exercise: We all know that taking a spin class, or getting in a swimming pool are not the wisest moves once you've had your embryo transfer, but gentle exercise is advisable, as it gets blood pumping around your whole body. So, taking a gentle walk, especially somewhere picturesque with low pollution is a great way to spend some time.

- Relax: It is so important to rest and relax as this helps to destress and keep cortisol (the stress hormone) at bay. It may sound incredibly simple, but reading a good book, watching a movie or doing an easy meditation are perfect ways to keep you relaxed and take some time for you.

- Create positive vibes: One of the loveliest things I heard that someone did in their 2WW, was to write a letter to the universe about why they wanted to be pregnant and have a baby. Creating positive vibes and reflecting on your dreams can be mentally positive. It worked for her so why not give it a go.

@iwannabemamabear

Support for men during the two-week wait

The two-week wait for women is a mix of emotions, from anxiety, worry and frustration. No one knows how they are going to be affected as they're focusing intensely on getting pregnant and having a baby – they cannot imagine the impact the process will have on them. For women trying to conceive, the shock of not being able to conceive naturally, and the struggle they have to even reach the point of the two-week wait has ramifications throughout their lives; their self-worth, their relationships with their partner, friends and family, and their working life. It's something I regularly hear, and offer help within my counselling service – providing coping mechanisms to survive the two-week wait and coming to terms with the trauma of the fertility experience.

However, I often wonder, 'What about the men on the two-week wait?'. What do men feel at this time? How are they coping with their emotions and the emotions and expectations of their partner? It's hard for a woman to describe her thoughts, feelings and physical emotions, so where would a man start?

From the beginning of the treatment men say it's all about their partner; on getting called into an appointment from the waiting room, it's naturally the partners name that's called. The doctor speaks directly to the partner, and the partner is offered support, not them.

Most support groups are for women and are full of women, so where can a man go for help? They are on this journey too. The men I have spoken with are wanting to support their partner and to make their partner happy. They focus more on their partner and forget to look after themselves, so when a man gets to the two-week wait, what should he do? Do they know they can contact the clinic and book in to see the counsellor for support on their own? Do they know where to get support from, who is there to help them, and if there is a support network outside of their relationship?

Everybody's journey is different. Not everyone feels the same and we often forget that feelings will change during different stages. Fertility treatment is an emotional rollercoaster for everyone involved. Sometimes, on reflection, when I've engaged with heterosexual couples, I wonder if the couple have reflected on the impact this will have on their relationship — how they'll cope together as a couple, and individually. Do men naively assume the journey won't affect them? Do they think the woman has a bigger part to play on this journey?

Sandra Bateman @nfs_hub

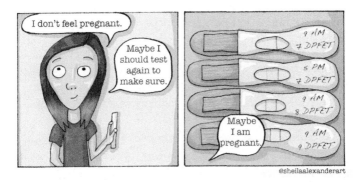

@sheilaalexanderart

There's so much emotional and financial pressure

I think that no matter how you get pregnant, the two-week wait can be a very strange experience. Two weeks, which normally go by pretty quickly, suddenly feels like an eternity. After IVF (in-vitro fertilisation) that two-week wait can be unbearable. There is so much more emotional and financial pressure riding on this period of time, and the result of the test at the end could change everything.

I took a few days off work after the transfer, to rest a little bit, but then went to work as normal to keep my mind busy and distracted. Obviously, thoughts filled my mind constantly of what might or might not be. You're advised to eat carefully, as though you are pregnant, and avoid exercise or being around too much stress. It's a funny limbo of acting pregnant just in case; you feel a bit of a fraud. A glass of wine would have really helped, but you can't take the risk.

It was recommended by a friend to listen to the Zita West meditation, which I downloaded every night. It isn't my normal sort of thing to do, but if nothing else, it reminded me to take it easy. And usually, I went into a pretty deep sleep whilst listening, so that was nice. It helped me to switch off from all the thoughts racing through my mind.

I also went to the cinema with my husband, went out for dinner. and enjoyed short walks to keep ourselves busy — and most importantly — not talk about infertility.

We told family, a few friends and a selection of colleagues about the IVF, so they knew it had happened, but we did ask them all not to talk about it. We really didn't want any extra pressure added to what we were already going through, and we also didn't want to get anyone's hopes up in case it didn't work. I deliberately didn't tell my Grandmother, because I didn't want to worry her.

The temptation to test early was insane, but, somehow, I managed to stop myself. I knew it could be a huge mistake; a false negative if taken too early, or it could just be negative, and I wasn't ready to hear that.

Three days before the end of the two-weeks (test day), it was our nephew's christening. I'd been asked to make cupcakes, which I happily agreed as I love to bake. I made three batches, each batch worse than the one before. I was normally really good at baking, but they just wouldn't rise and tasted horrible. I burst into tears and called my sister-in-law to apologise. I promised to pick up some nice cakes from Waitrose on the way to the christening. I couldn't stop crying about my failure though; I was so upset with myself. It was at that point when I was in the bathroom drying my eyes that I thought…

hang on a minute…what… no, this isn't like me… surely not… maybe?

I reached for the pregnancy test kit, which I had carefully hidden out of sight on the top shelf in the bathroom. I knew I was a few days early, but it felt like something had changed in me, and these tears had come from nowhere. I did the test and remember shaking as I waited for the result; I even turned the test over, so I didn't just stare at it. When it was time, I carefully turned the test over and held my breath…I looked down and there it was… my big fat POSITIVE.

"PETER, PETER… PETER!" I shouted, as I ran down the stairs, and he was standing in the living room ironing his shirt, "You'll never guess what…"

Lianne Baker, UK

Thoughts on the two-week wait (2WW)

Ask any woman or man what words they associate with the two-week wait (2WW) and you'll hear the following:

- The dreaded two week wait

- The hardest part of treatment

- The longest few days of my life.

So, why is this time really so tough? I personally endured five sets of two-week waits during the six years of fertility treatment, and each time was incredibly difficult, regardless of what the treatment itself had been like.

For me, I think the act of stopping any real activity, such as clinic visits, scans etc, meant an inevitable time of self-focus, and with that, over analysis of every twinge or ache I was feeling, or worse, lack of any twinge or ache. It's almost impossible to switch off and this is my first point.

- Don't expect the impossible: by this I don't mean anything to do with outcome and everything to do with attitude. This time is almost inevitably going to be hard as you walk the tightrope between hope and fear, so rather than beating yourself up for having these feelings, identify them as normal and reasonable responses to a difficult situation. Knowing this will serve you much better.

- Secondly, from a place of self-compassion and honesty, take action to help yourself through this time. Put in place anything and everything that will help you to manage this period.

    If you are able to forward plan some strategies, so much the better, but take time to think what could be helpful for you. This will vary hugely from one person to the next, so it's important to pause and reflect on what you specifically need. For me, it was to provide some form of daily framework that would enable me, conversely, to let go a little. So, I would make sure I was doing something physical, something nourishing, and something informative each day.

    I would book in to meet with a few trusted friends that I could be myself with, and I would treat myself as I would my best friend – and expect only what I was able to give.

- Lastly, I would say be flexible in your expectations. It may be that one day you chose to be incredibly sociable as a distraction technique and a way to connect with a wider sense of self. On other days, you may need to retreat and recover, and that's perfect too. You may not know until the day itself, so hold flexibility and self-awareness as a key part of your coping strategy.

As a final point there have been patients I have known over the years who've said they definitely were able to tell that they were pregnant during the two-week wait. However, I would say they are in the minority, and this definitely wasn't my experience. In fact, the two times I 'knew' fertility treatment hadn't worked were when it had, and I was in fact pregnant! The symptoms, or lack of them, for me, were so often confused with the effects of the progesterone I was taking, that it was almost impossible for me to guess what the outcome would be.

On that note, and as an aside, the two times I was pregnant after treatment were the least orthodox of the 2WW experiences. The first was after ten days at the Edinburgh fringe festival and the second at the end of a trip to Euro Disney, where I ended up self-injecting in Disney toilets ... totally surreal!

It is this reality that best points to one of the hardest realisations about the 2WW – that there is an unknown aspect to the science and to our own best efforts. We may well have ticked every box, done all we could do, and had a 'perfect' cycle, (whatever that is), but the 2WW ultimate life lesson is that there will always be a part of fertility treatment that is beyond our control, and even out of the control of the best scientists.

What we are left with is hope, and that perhaps is the hardest of all emotions to feel, and hold onto, somewhat precariously, during the 2WW.

Anya Sizer Twitter @sizeranya

From worrier to warrior

When navigating a fertility journey and particularly the two-week wait, there is so much to think about, consider and quite frankly – worry about!

It doesn't have to be that way though. I teach my IVF coaching clients to adapt an 80/20 rule. 80% of their time they endeavour to live their life, and 20% of their time is for thinking, researching and worrying. However, to do this you need to train your brain to worry when you want to, and not allow worrying to be the boss of you. My coaching tool: 'From Worrier to Warrior' is a firm favourite with my clients. This tool not only takes charge of your worries, but it helps you take action to deal with your worries and embrace the 80/20 rule.

1. **Build a habit of deliberate worry**

   Choose a place that you intend to spend your time worrying in each day. This could be a worry chair or a particular room (never the bedroom). Come to this place at a set time each day to worry/research/think. By doing so, you are training your mind to understand that YOU are in charge and your worries are not the boss of you. You're not suppressing your worries, simply postponing them until you are ready.

2. **Create a worry list**

   In your worry place, get onto paper all the things that are troubling you, but also write down any research you may need to do, or actions you might need to take. Take a few minutes to free write and don't judge your thoughts. Crazy is good!

3. **Categorise your worries**

   Use a traffic light system to organise your worries:

   Green Worries – worries that need to be solved and are immediate and pressing. There's evidence that what you are worried about is true.

To overcome 'Green Worries' you need to ACT. Make a decision on what you need to do, set a deadline and do it! Don't procrastinate, as action needs to be taken to remove this worry.

Amber Worries – worries that are imaginary – the 'what if's'. It's likely that you'll have a lot of these. These are worries about a future event that you may or may not be able to control.

To overcome 'Amber Worries' you need to plan. Start devising an action plan to ease this worry. You can include things that you need to research or questions you need to ask. Stick to your plan to move forward with this worry.

Red Worries – worries that you cannot control or answer. Red worries include worrying about what someone else might think, feel, say or do.

To overcome 'Red Worries' embrace uncertainty and know that you are not responsible for other people and cannot control their actions or thoughts.

Learning to take back control of your worries takes time. The more you can practice, the easier and more natural it will become. Remember, fertility is part of you, as is the two-week wait, but by no means all of you. And, now, is the time to start living your life.

Kate Davies @your_fertility_journey

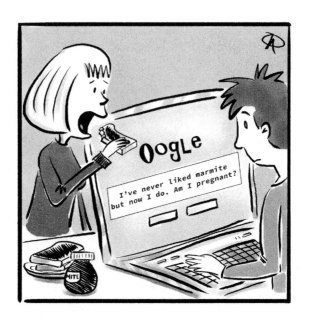

Try something new in your two-week wait (TWW)

My husband and I lived a very adventurous life and travelled as much as we could. We learned to mountain bike, salsa dance, surf, wakeboard, snowboard and explored many different beautiful places. We took our fertility for granted, and thought we had plenty of time. Just before our wedding, I got pregnant, but sadly it ended too soon; our first miscarriage. At the time I believed there was a plan, and that it wasn't our time. Five months after our wedding, I was pregnant again. It was perfect and surely was meant to be this time, right? Unfortunately, this pregnancy also ended in a miscarriage.

So, now it seemed there could be an issue. We ended up seeing a fertility specialist, and a year later began our first IUI (intra-uterine insemination) cycle. This was so different from my previous experiences, when I didn't realize I was pregnant until I was 'late'. Now I was prepping my body, monitoring everything, injecting myself with medications and inviting another man (our doctor) into the room to help impregnate me. Wait-what! This was not how I pictured our special moment. I wasn't sure what to expect during the much talked about 'two-week wait' (TWW). I had a very busy career and thought I would just throw myself into work, and it would be no different than any other week. How wrong could I be!

I wasn't ready for the anxious feelings, the obsessing over every 'symptom' in my body, and the rollercoaster of emotions I felt due to the hormones. I couldn't help my obsession with wanting to take a pregnancy test every day! I also wasn't prepared for having to give up the activities my husband and I did on a regular basis. This was pretty devastating to me. I don't know why I didn't know this, but I was shocked. We couldn't even travel to our favorite destination to get away for a break, due to its altitude. I realized quickly that this wasn't going to be as easy as I thought it would be. I decided I needed to focus on something else and try not to stress ALL day and ALL night long.

One activity that wasn't restricted was yoga. So, I researched and found a pregnancy yoga program that could work during this period and help me develop a good habit for the duration of my pregnancy – if the IUI worked. I also thought it could be a great addition to my current fun activities.

Well, much to my surprise, I fell in love with the pregnancy yoga videos. They were really helpful and provided me with a different level of peace during the rest of my two-week wait. I had to really focus, and I was forced to think only about my breathing and movements. What I wasn't expecting was how impactful it was on my mind throughout the day. I looked forward to the morning routine and found my mood was lifted. I also started sleeping better. What a win!

When this pregnancy also ended in a miscarriage, I was incredibly grateful to have yoga to help me heal, emotionally and physically. During my next IUI and subsequent pregnancy (yay!).

I was on bedrest for two months and yoga was one of the few approved activities I could participate in for the duration of that pregnancy. I continued my yoga program until the day I went into labor. All of these benefits that impacted my mind, body and spirit were due to me taking a chance and trying something new.

I wanted to share this, not to tell everyone to take up yoga specifically, but to encourage you to try something new during your two-week wait. Beginning a new physical hobby has so many benefits, including:

- building confidence as you learn something new

- reducing stress by changing the chemicals in your body, and

- focusing your mind on something positive outside of your fertility journey.

These are benefits you definitely need while you are in the TWW. You also never know when or how this new activity could help you in the future.

I'm sending you hugs and positive thoughts for your journey. You can do this!

Jackie Figueras @thesupportivemama

The two-week wait is a rough but wondrous ride

As someone who likes to be prepared, my first IVF, (in vitro fertilisation) embryo transfer happened somewhat suddenly and unexpectedly. During the ovarian stimulation and egg retrieval process, I developed OHSS (ovarian hyper stimulation syndrome), which can be life threatening. When I went in for a check-up on embryo transfer day, I was convinced the doctors would take a "freeze all, transfer later" approach – meaning I wouldn't have an embryo transferred today. However, that's not what happened. Within ten minutes of walking through the door, I had my very first embryo transfer. After handing me an instruction sheet with four bullet points: don't take baths, don't exercise, etc, the clinicians told me to continue with my life as normal, and take a home pregnancy test in fourteen days. Before I even realized what had happened, my husband and I were in the car on our way home, and for probably the first time in my life, I was PUPO (pregnant until proven otherwise), and thrown right into the depths of the "IVF two-week wait."

Those two weeks were a rough but wondrous ride, where I experienced the highest of highs and the lowest of lows – an internal battle between horrific anxiety and newfound, unbridled hope.

The single most important thing that kept me sane was the support and love from my husband, family, friends, and strangers from around the world – my incredible online support network who helped keep my spirits up when the weight of my circumstances crushed me. Reading encouraging stories on Instagram, watching IVF success videos on YouTube, and listening to infertility podcasts, all helped me find my positive pants on even the darkest of days.

During this emotional period, I tried to live as healthily as possible, by preparing nutritious meals and spending time outside, as nature helped calm me down and regain my strength. Still, there were times when the anxiety became too overwhelming and the fear of a failed cycle unbearable. In those moments, distraction was key. Refocusing my thoughts and redirecting my attention to a TV show, movie, game or book offered temporary relief from IVF and infertility worries.

I'm not going to lie, I did what probably most people going through a two-week wait do, regardless of what the clinics tell you - I symptom spotted and consulted Dr. Google. If you want to keep your sanity, I recommend you don't. But, if you're like me and just can't help yourself, here's a tip: set a timer. Allow yourself a certain amount of time to analyze your pinches and cramping abdomen, but then stop. Distract yourself. Don't let it consume you, because once you go down that road, it's hard to turn back. Plus, whatever you feel can be a good or bad sign – there's just no real way to tell.

Unfortunately, for me, this transfer and the two frozen transfers that followed weren't successful. Surprisingly, as difficult and nerve-wracking as each of the two-week waits were, I also enjoyed some of it. For the first time in my life, I knew that I was carrying life, that this tiny ball of cells in my uterus might become our future son or daughter. No one can ever take those moments of joy away from me. We'll keep going, and maybe one day I will go through a TWW, not PUPO, but PASP – pregnant and staying pregnant.

Kate @hopematters.always

What I recall from the horrible TWW

- I wasn't working and was at home with nothing to do, but worry. Every IVF cycle I did, I was anxious throughout the TWW, constantly thinking, 'Am I pregnant?' I'm sure this is normal. IVF worked eventually, so the worry didn't impact the outcome.

- I made sure to spend time with people who knew nothing of what I was going through for maximum distraction. That helped to lift a few hours of the day.

- I painted the study. Not sure how advisable that was, but it was during the cycle that actually worked! My daughter is about to turn sixteen. If your embies are going to stick and hang on in there, they will do so, whatever you do.

- I lurked on chat rooms, but I never joined in. I lingered on the posts of those who were buoyant and moved swiftly on from those with sad news.

- I felt my boobs constantly, embarrassingly so once in a restaurant! If they 'buzzed' I was happy! On our first cycle they suddenly stopped buzzing ...

Diane Chandler, Author of *Moondance*

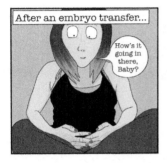 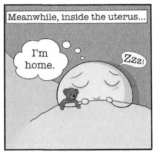

@sheilaalexanderart

Excerpts from the book *336 hours*

Day 3

09.05am

It's good news, Steve said hurriedly. (Phew, phew, phew – thank you, embryos; thank you, Steve; THANK YOU, GOD!) Three of our five embryos are looking strong, with the remaining two possible, and still developing ... just a little more slowly. So, with no standout winner just yet, the doctor said he'd like to culture them for a couple more days in the lab and aim for a blastocyst transfer on day five.

A blastocyst, even though it sounds like something you'd find orbiting the solar system, or something a teenager might wake up to erupting from the end of her nose, is actually the one thing that everyone hopes to achieve in this game.

But one thing DH and I have learnt over the last couple of

years is that assessing embryos is a complex task. And we have always found it disconcerting to watch the number of seemingly viable embryos decline as the days pass by. Initially, we had assumed that every embryo equals a baby, but sadly, this is far from being the case.

Day 5 – 2.20pm

There's a certain walk reserved for a very limited range of situations in life. It's the walk I'll be walking for the rest of today, and it reveals to everyone around me, one of several possibilities:

I'm a drug mule, rectally smuggling huge quantities of cocaine into the country.

I've just suddenly and catastrophically soiled my underwear.

I'm going through IVF and have just had my eggs collected or...

I'm going through IVF and have just had my embryos transferred.

In each of these scenarios (I'm imagining, of course, as I've only actually experienced three of them), a woman is seen taking miniature, shuffling steps forwards, her back rigid, her buttocks clenched, a look of wild panic and yet intense concentration betraying the frantic internal dialogue that's taking place inside her head.

The final two IVF-related walks are actually very similar; during the first one (after egg collection), a woman is physically unable to walk, and during the second, (after her embaby is transferred) she's simply too scared of the effects of gravity to stand up and walk out of the clinic. It might make no sense whatsoever, but I feel that our embryos are so delicately balanced within my body that they might drop out at any second. I feel that if I were to hop, skip, slip over, cough, sneeze, blow my nose or even fart in an over-zealous fashion, they would be expelled from my vagina instantaneously.

Logically, I know this can't happen, and I also know that our transfer was 'textbook perfect' – well, as perfect as an embryo transfer could ever be, that is.

Day 9 – 11.30am

Nat has tentatively enquired a couple of times now about how I'm feeling, and I've tried my best to answer her question, whilst also trying to protect her from the full contents of my head.

Having had a total absence of 'symptoms' for the last twenty-four hours, I did, around thirty minutes ago, experience a couple of sharp stomach cramps, which have simultaneously filled me with immense hope and utter despair.

I wondered if the cramps were a sign that Kenneth and Donaghy are busy implanting into my womb as we speak, or, if, alternatively, they're a sign that they've stopped developing altogether, and my womb is getting ready to turn itself inside out as soon as I stop taking the pessaries in a few days' time.

Or maybe it's the pessaries themselves that are causing those brief, niggly cramps.

Or maybe the cramps aren't even real; perhaps they're just a figment of my imagination, fuelled only by my desperate desire to rustle up some sort of pregnancy-confirming evidence.

Day 12 – 11.30am

It seems the inevitable 'toilet terror' which accompanies every IVF two-week wait has begun in earnest today.

My period is due in two days' time, but I know that if the pessaries don't keep it at bay, and there's nothing exciting like a pregnancy to stop it in its tracks, then those tell-tale spots of blood could be making an appearance any time now.

Each time I venture to the bathroom for a pee, I have to counsel myself to stand up, wipe and whip the toilet paper up plainly in front of my eyes to confront any tinges of colour that may be present.

I wonder how many more toilet trips I will need to make before our official test date. Far too many for comfort. I know that for certain.

I've found myself talking to Kenneth and Donaghy a lot today, and asking them to send me a signal that they're still alive, and that they're managing to hang on in there somehow.

What's causing my distinctly not-pregnant feelings, I'd like to know. Is it an instinctive acknowledgement that it really is time to start grieving the loss of our genetic children? Or are these feelings only a manifestation of my own worst fears?

I keep reminding myself that fear is a powerful emotion and that it's only human nature to dread the disappearance of the people and things that we want and need the most.

But what I'm sensing in the middle of my stomach, the nothingness that is permeating my body from the womb outwards, feels both distressingly real and heartsinkingly familiar.

I fear it's more than just the fear that's talking to me now.

Rachel Cathan – author

Making your two-week wait one of laughter and happiness

'Exciting and complete torture' is how the two-week wait (TWW) has been described to me, on more than one occasion. However, the fact that you are at this point is a fantastic achievement. Your embryo is now safely where it can thrive, and your expectations of success should be high.

As you will have been told, all you need to do now is:

- continue to eat well,

- stay hydrated,

- get enough sleep

- relax and remain positive!

The first three points are easy enough, but I know the last two can be challenging. They are, however, important, because in Chinese Medicine, feelings of stress or negativity can be detrimental to fertility. This is because these emotions constrict the flow of energy in your body – for example, you may have noticed you get tight shoulders when stressed. Constricting the energy flow is similar to setting up a contraflow on the motorway – the traffic/energy soon backs up and creates a blockage.

By contrast, when you're relaxed and positive there are no obstacles – your energy can flow freely. This free flow of energy to the uterus is beneficial to your fertility, as it creates a receptive and welcoming environment for the embryo.

Whilst this is all very well in theory, trying to relax and be positive can often have the opposite effect. Therefore, I hope these tips help:

- Acupuncture

  I always recommend acupuncture treatment pre and post transfer, and again the week after transfer – it is hugely relaxing and increases blood flow to the uterus to support implantation.

  Its efficacy alongside ART (assisted reproductive treatment), is supported by numerous studies. One study[1] found that acupuncture before and after IVF (in-vitro fertilisation) nearly doubled the chance of success compared to those who simply underwent IVF.

- Laughter

  When we laugh our body relaxes, we feel more positive and our energy flows. However, it can be tricky to laugh on demand, so let someone else do the work! I ask my patients to download a selection of their favourite comedies so that after embryo transfer, they can go home, relax and allow someone else to make them laugh. Watch comedies after transfer and often during the TWW.

There is a study[2] to back this up too. It found that a visit from a therapeutic medical clown immediately after embryo transfer increased the rate of pregnancy to 36%, compared with 20% for women whose embryo transfer was comedy-free. (Therapeutic medical clowning is also known as 'hospital clowning' or 'clown doctors').

- Happiness A-Z

  If you catch yourself thinking negatively – don't panic. You won't have caused any damage, but try and steer yourself back towards happiness. One way to do this is to work through the alphabet from A-Z, and for each letter think of something that makes you smile. This is a great exercise to do at bedtime.

- Photo album

  Create a 'happiness album' of twenty to thirty photos on your phone; pictures that make you smile. They can be of anything as long as they give you a warm, happy feeling. Whenever you are feeling a little low, take a look at them. You'll be surprised at how easy it is to change the focus of your thoughts and bring yourself back to a happy, positive place.

- Believe

  Never underestimate the power of your mind. Hundreds of studies demonstrate how our thoughts can influence our bodies – both positively and negatively. It is vital to believe that you will succeed – have faith and jump in with both feet!

  Practising affirmations can really help create a positive mind set. Create your own personal affirmation along the lines of: 'I am happy, healthy and fertile'. Phrasing must be positive and stated in the present tense as the subconscious doesn't understand past or future, only the present moment. If it's stated in the future as in: 'I'm looking forward to being pregnant,' it can remain there … just out of your reach. So, instead say: "I am enjoying my healthy pregnancy".

Choose a phrase that is simple, positive and productive to your situation. Say it aloud when you're on your own, or in your head if out and about. Repeat it at least twenty times a day and then visualise yourself as pregnant and blooming. Initially this may feel awkward, but the more you practise it, the more natural it becomes, and the more you will trust it.

- Visualisation

  Place your hands flat over your lower abdomen, breathe deeply and picture your uterus as a big fluffy duvet; a warm, welcoming and wonderful place where your embryo can snuggle in and grow.

I wish you every success and happiness!

Justine Hankin @justinehankin

[1] https://www.ncbi.nlm.nih.gov/pubmed/11937123

[2] https://www.ncbi.nlm.nih.gov/pubmed/21211796

A two-week wait story

Corrine and Jack are halfway through their fourth IVF cycle. Jack likes to say she's having IVF. She says they are having IVF. They need IVF because they both have problems. Jack's got very poor swimmers – that's what they call sperm on the fertility web forum, and she has problems releasing an egg – Anovulatory cycles. Corrine is through the down regulation phase of IVF and has just finished the stimulation medication.

'Thank God that bit's over. It's not easy living with a 'down-regulated' woman,' Jack sighs in the kitchen of their terraced house in Box, Wiltshire.

Corrine sits at the kitchen table with a small packet in front of her. She reaches into her medication bag to find a needle for the injection. Jack's face is pale with dark shadows under his eyes. He's handsome, broad shouldered and lean. She knows he looks tired as she unwraps the box. It's the trigger injection to ripen her eggs. She's relieved to have finished the stimulation medication, thankful for her ovary's performance; once again it looks as though she has produced plenty of eggs.

For the last twelve days, she's been counting her follicles, reporting their growth, millimetre by millimetre on the forum that supports her and thousands of other women during the IVF process. She calls them her 'invisible friends'. Corrine thinks of the many traps along the IVF journey as she draws the fluid up from the vial into the syringe. Poor ovarian response. Overstimulation. Early ovulation. The steel shaft of the needle glimmers in the remnants of September's evening's light. She taps the syringe to remove the air bubble, picks up the needle still in its packet and walks across the kitchen's oak floor, into the hallway and stands on a brown wool rug in front of the full-length mirror. She unwraps the needle and fixes it to the syringe and pulls her jeans down to her knees. She pinches flesh from the outer top of her left thigh, noticing cellulite where she once had none. There are small scabs marking previous injection sites, and two bruises where the jabs went amiss. She inserts the needle into her thigh and pushes down on the syringe. It stings and her eyes flicker. Then she takes the needle out of her skin, pulls her jeans back up and fastens her leather belt.

From across the hallway, Jack notices how bloated Corrine's abdomen is, and how worried she looks, as she dismantles the injection, snaps off the needle and puts it inside a yellow sharps box on top of the table in the hallway. If IVF doesn't work, it will take three or four months for Corrine to recover. With failure, Jack knows her hopes will be squashed and she'll be anxious and stressed. If they get a positive pregnancy test, he worries about it going wrong, like it did last time. It's taken many months for Corrine to look him in the eye without tears. He felt they shouldn't try again so soon; she wasn't ready, but she was insistent, so he couldn't say no. He knows he could lose her again …

Jack walks to the fridge, grabs a bottle of cider and opens it. Corrine can't drink and he misses their evenings in by the fire with a glass of red wine. He looks at her, 'Elderflower?'

'Why don't you have one with me?' she replies.

'I fancy a cider.' He pours the bottle of cider into a long glass and sits down at the kitchen table.

Corrine looks at him disapprovingly as she walks back into the kitchen, 'Do you have to drink?'

'One won't hurt.'

'Don't forget you have to produce your sample.'

'How could I forget?'

Corrine looks away from him as she sits down. Jack gets the cordial and a bottle of fizzy water out of the fridge. He makes the elderflower drink and hands it to Corrine, 'Is that it with the jabs now until the op?'

'Yup, jab free day tomorrow.'

'Cool, I'll make us a nice lunch then. We can stay in and get an early night. What time do we have to be at the clinic?'

'Six.'

'That's early.'

'Yup, first on the list.'

Jack walks back to the table and sits down next to his wife. He leans in towards her and grabs her hand. 'God, I hope it works this time. I worry about you.'

Corrine cuts him off. 'Don't worry about me, I'll be ok. What's important is that we're trying.'

'Yeah, but what if?'

'We both have to hope.'

'I do, but I'm scared about you if…'

Corrine cuts across again, 'Don't say it, please, don't'…

'Ok, darling', Jack reaches for her, 'Come here.'

Jack and Corrine kiss just once, then Corrine rests her head on his shoulder and keeps her eyes closed.

Five days later, inside the clinic embryo transfer suite, everything looks dazzling white – the walls, the comfy chairs, and the carpet – and the room smells of hospital disinfectant.

Corrine climbs onto the bed with stirrups. She feels steel, cold against her skin. Jack holds her hand, he is gowned, hair covered in a round plastic blue cap and he wears plastic wraps on his shoes. He pretends to be a doctor, moves to the front of Corrine and stretches his gloved fingers between Corrine's legs and laughs.

'Don't…behave.'

The door opens and the doctor enters. Jack looks down and moves quickly back to Corrine's side.

'Hello, I'm Doctor Poloni.'

'Hello'. Jack waves his hand.

The doctor tightens the stirrups around Corrine's legs as the chair elevates and extra lights are turned on to guide the placement of the embryos.

'Okay, comfortable? Are you ready?'

Corrine nods, 'Yes, I'm ready'.

The doctor turns to Jack. 'How about you?'

Jack smiles. 'Ready as I'll ever be.'

The doctor's masked face draws close between the top of Corrine's thighs as he brings the catheter towards him. Jack looks away sharply as though he has been slapped. He shuffles on his feet and coughs. Corrine's bladder feels like a ball pressing up inside her. She's worried she might lose control. She turns to look at Jack and taps his hand. 'Don't make me laugh.'

'Why, might you spring a leak?' Jack teases.

The doctor looks up at them with a smile. 'This won't take long and you need a full bladder for correct placement.'

'I'll hold on.' Corrine sighs as she fights to control bladder muscles and not think of the indignity of it all. She breathes deep, squirms and controls her bladder as the catheter penetrates up into her womb. It hurts. She breathes deeply as she feels the fabric of the bench on the underside of her thighs and focuses on the white lights on the ceiling. After ten uneasy minutes with the catheter in place and the doctor's head between her legs with Jack by her side, holding her hand, their embryos are safely inside.

'There, we're done, both in the best position.'

'Great'.

The doctor removes the catheter. Corrine tries not to look at it as he takes it to the embryologist in the lab, who inspects it and then returns confirming it's empty. The doctor switches off the extra lighting. 'You need to stay here for ten minutes. I'll leave you with the nurse. She'll explain your medication. Good luck.'

Corrine's legs are released from the stirrups and she lies on the chair with her legs together, pulling the gown down as much as she can.

Later in the changing area, she dresses and struggles to get comfortable in her clothes. Swollen and sore from the egg collection, she wriggles her bum to get into her jeans. She squeezes in enough to fasten the zip. Jack sits down beside her, careful not to get too close. He knows she's still tender. A nurse pulls the screen aside.

'Is everything OK?'

'Yeah.'

'Good. No baths and no sex for two weeks.'

'I wouldn't call that good.' Jack winks at Corrine.

On their way out of the clinic, they collect the progesterone injections, and then walk in the sunshine towards their car. Inside, Corrine tilts her seat slightly back, and Jack starts the engine, pulling out of the car park as smoothly as he can. Corrine leans back with her eyes closed throughout the drive home. They don't speak much through the two-hour journey.

When they are back in the kitchen, Jack stands near the table in front of the medicine bag. He holds a small glass vial, breaks the top off, puts it in the sharps box and places a large thick needle onto the syringe. Then he draws the liquid up into the syringe.

'Which cheek tonight?' He turns and wiggles his bum at Corrine.

'Right'. Corrine's fists are curled tight.

'Turn around then'.

Corrine closes her eyes and drops her jeans and the top of her French knickers. As she does so, Jack pinches her left buttock gently, 'Your turn tomorrow'.

Corrine frowns, she hates these injections. Jack has to do them as she can't reach. They are intramuscular, in that, they go deep into the muscle, and the needle is huge. She has to have one every day for the next two weeks until test day, 'Don't, please just get on with it.'

'Do you want the numbing cream?'

'Please.'

Jack's finger is raised over her right buttock slick with the cream. Neither of them speaks as they wait for it to take effect. The safety cap still covers the needle as Jack keeps the syringe warm in his hand. Its oil base is easier to insert into flesh if warm. If it's cold it makes Corrine's bum lumpy and she has even more problems sitting down. Jack unsheathes the needle and when Corrine's not expecting it, he jabs the thick needle right into the flesh of the outer park of her right buttock. It's quick. He's learnt that surprise is the best tactic and the 1.5 inch needle glides all the way in. He presses the syringe down, but it takes a while to go in, and he feels slightly sick as he watches the liquid disappear. Corrine is silent, her fingers start to relax once he removes the needle from her flesh, but blood pools at the injection site. 'It's a bleeder,' Jack says. He reaches for a ball of cotton wool to stem the flow and holds it there until it stops.

After the injection, Corrine retreats to the sofa in their living room. She sits down very carefully and switches on her laptop, logging into the fertility web forum to announce that she has two eight cell 'embies' on board. Virtual friends offer congratulations and share tales of relief of getting this far as so many don't. She can breathe now and try to relax into her two-week wait until test day. The two-week wait is the worst when endless whirlpools of thought make her ponder every twinge as a sign of pregnancy. Her hands feel the lower part of her belly, still puffy from the drugs. She knows it will take weeks to go down, but hope is rising that this time her belly might start to grow. Maybe this time she will get past fourteen weeks. She logs out of the forum and looks through online maternity catalogues.

The day after, Corrine tidies the old cupboard drawer in her
bedside cabinet. She sees a pink bar of soap, shaped as a heart.
It's been kept in her bedroom drawer for nearly seventeen
years, a remnant from her 21st birthday from an old boyfriend,
Michael. She picks it up. Two halves open to reveal a white key
in the middle. She looks down at it and feels the decades flicker
past. Why has she had to wait so long for motherhood? Michael
has three children; the eldest is already fifteen. It's not fair. Just
not fair.

Corrine pads from her bedroom and into the bathroom where
she turns the sink tap on and plunges the heart-shaped soap
under the running water. She lathers her hands, washing clean
her jealousy, dissolving all the issues that were once between
them. She turns the taps off and discards the soggy, misshapen
soap in the sink. In front of the bathroom shelves she stares
at the duo packet of pregnancy tests. Picking up one packet,
she turns it over, eyes flicking over the text. She doesn't need
to read it. She's read it a million times before. Pausing, she puts
the pregnancy test back with a quick dart of her hand. She
can't, not yet. It's not time. She's promised herself she won't test
early. She mustn't this time. There's still two weeks to wait. Two
weeks. And they have only just begun.

Justine Bold @justinebold

How I spent my two-week wait

I had acupuncture after my embryo transfer. I'd been having
it ahead of and during my treatment and believe it had a
significant impact on my treatment, so I was keen to continue
post transfer. The day after my embryo transfer, hubby and I
went to the Suffolk coast to a little cottage. I knew we needed to
get away and I wanted us to be by the water. He'd planned some
yummy food, as he's the cook in our relationship, and we spent

a few days walking, talking, sleeping and just being together, away from everything. There was no wi-fi, no TV. I remember, we watched 'The Secret' on my iPad as I'd downloaded it. We talked about everything, but what was actually going on. It gave us both a bit of headspace, before returning to work a few days later.

For the following week and a half, I made a point of seeing some friends, going for walks, doing yoga … just trying to keep busy. It wasn't too awful to be honest, as I continued to live my life. I also made a point of doing visualisations, especially whilst in the shower, as my friend said I should imagine washing my pregnant tummy, which I did. Did my visualisations work? Well I guess so! We were lucky and had a positive pregnancy test after our first attempt.

Natalie Silverman @fertilitypoddy

My top tips for your two-week wait (TWW)

The TWW feels like the longest two weeks of your entire life. Mine was only nine days, but it felt like nine years, and I'm sure I looked nine years older by the end. These are my top tips for surviving:

1. Stay away from Dr Google. During my TWW, I tried my best not to Google anything. Any symptoms that I had, I put straight down to the progesterone pessaries, to save myself worrying whether the embryo had implanted.

2. Keep busy. When we were undergoing IVF (in-vitro fertilisation), I had my egg transfer in the morning, and then went back to work in the afternoon. I found that keeping busy was key to maintaining my focus, and not letting worries or doubts kick in. On my days off, I found myself falling down the Dr Google rabbit hole (a big no-no, see above), and obsessing over the tiniest things. So, for me it was better to be working. I also discovered

crossword puzzles – such a great distraction, as they give you a focus and engage your mind. My worst enemy was my overthinking mind!

3. Find your tribe. Find people you can talk to who really 'get it'. Unfortunately, unless people have struggled with trying to conceive, or undergone IVF, they simply don't and cannot understand what it's like. This is obviously through no fault of theirs, as why would they understand if they haven't been exposed to it? I've found the Instagram community to be completely invaluable. The wonderful women on there are the kindest, more supportive people, who truly 'get it'.

4. Take back control. Do whatever you feel is necessary to regain a little bit of power in what can seem like a never-ending uphill struggle. Whether that is exercising, meditating, making copious notes and lists, cooking lots of nutritious food, or like me, throwing away every single piece of plastic that you own. Whatever is it, indulge yourself. Ultimately IVF is completely out of your control, as is much of life, so it can help to feel like you have an influence over something.

5. Don't give up. This may not be the case for everyone, but my husband and I decided from the very beginning, that under no circumstances would we give up. Even though it's a hard and long journey, we promised each other that we won't stop until we get our family. I kept that in the forefront of my mind during our TWW, so that if the result was negative, I knew it wasn't the end.

Sophie Martin @the.infertile.midwife

Excerpt from the book *Warrior*

19 August 2015

Day 18

The transfer has happened, so I'm now technically pregnant!
Bit of a curve ball on the call this morning – neither of the two
stronger embryos had quite made it to blastocyst stage. They
are 'morulas', which is one step behind. One was looking strong
and the other not quite as much, so the upshot is – they were
both put in. They only freeze blastocysts, so if it hadn't gone
in, it would have been discarded, so it was worth a shot. I could
end up with twins, but I'd take two over none, any day! So, there
we are. We made it to the final step of the procedure and now
the challenging two-week wait starts.

I don't know what I was expecting, but the transfer consisted
of the embryos being put in what was essentially a long, thin,
floppy straw, which was popped through my cervix (it didn't
hurt). The embryos were then pushed out. I mean, imagine
if they'd dropped out of the 'straw' on the way from the lab
to my 'lady area'? (Sorry, I can't say the 'v' word, I'm British.)
Presumably they've thought it through and the straw is safe, so
we'll say no more about it.

So, two embryos are inside me – glued inside me – and it's my
job to nurture them so they grow and thrive. I feel calm. It's
very exciting, and of course I really hope it works. But I also
have in mind that if it doesn't, we'll try again, and I believe one
of the times it will. I know what to expect now, and while I
wouldn't choose to do it all again, I know I won't be as anxious
about all the injections. Here's to staying calm and keeping busy!

22 August 2015

Day 21

The embryos have been inside me for four days now and I've
had a lot of period-like cramps, particularly during last night

and this morning. I'm finding it hard to stay positive as it feels so similar to all the other months when I haven't been pregnant. I don't know what the feeling is – it could be a side effect of the progesterone pessaries, or it could be implantation pain. I don't know what it is. My mind wants to work it out, so it uses past experiences to jump to conclusions about the future. These are just thoughts, not reality. I won't know until I take that test in nine days' time. That's the difficult part. I'm trying to fill my time and keep busy, but I'm bored. I'm glad to be going back to work on Monday. I hope I'll be busy.

We've been off work for two weeks now and not done that much other than go back and forth to the clinic, so we're both starting to get a bit fed up. Trying not to be stressed is stressful. I need something to do, people to see. The only people who are available to do something at short notice are those with babies or children, and Craig doesn't want me to see them in case I get catch an illness. I can't even go for a run or to the gym as it's not advised at this point. Argh, I need an outlet! It does make me grateful for my job. I'd go insane if I always had this much free time. I need stimulation, I need to use my brain and I need to exercise. I might slip out by myself, take a book and go get a coffee somewhere.

24 August 2015

Day 23

I went back to work today, and I feel better for having a sense of purpose and something to occupy myself with. Saturday was rough. I felt irritable and tearful all day.

I'm still having period pain quite a lot. I'm trying to work out if it's anything different from any other month, and I think it's probably a bit worse than usual. It feels like it does the day before my period, rather than a week before. I can console myself with that – perhaps something is different – although part of me is steeling myself for disappointment now. My mind is racing ahead to plan when we can try again and which deal to go for. I know I shouldn't, but I feel better when I know what my next move is. I shouldn't give up on the little embryos inside me though. For all I know, they're growing and thriving, while I've already written them off.

I said part of me was steeling myself for disappointment, but the other half is still hopeful and positive. Even though, as I'm writing this, I have such familiar period pain, I won't allow my thoughts to tell me that's definitely what it is. They're thoughts, not facts.

Earlier today, when I got in from work, Craig asked me to lie down with him on the bed. He never does that.

'Why?' I ask.

'Can't I give my pregnant wife a cuddle and make sure she's OK?'

I smile, despite wanting to tell him not to say that … not to tempt fate.

'How are they doing?'

'I don't know,' I say, honestly.

'You keep growing in there,' he says to the potential babies in my belly, stroking my belly gently. I take his hand and squeeze it. He wants this as much as I do.

One week till test day!

26 August 2015

Day 25

Five days until the test. That's hardly any time, and yet also an eternity away. I've still got period pain. My belly looks bloated and swollen. It's rounded low down and does look a bit like a pregnancy bump. That makes me excited. I read today that it's common to be bloated and look pregnant days after conception, so I really could be! I've never seen my belly stick out like that in such a rounded shape before. It's definitely something different to normal. It could be a side effect of the medication, but I read the leaflet (at least six times) and it didn't mention bloating.

I'm feeling the period-like cramps now and tuning in to analyse if they are different. I think they might be more on one side, which could mean embryos implanting. Eek, I could be pregnant! I'm excited for test day, but also dreading it. I don't know how I'll dare go through with it. I might wee on myself.

27 August 2015

Day 26

Four days until test day. I can't bear it. I'd say, I can't bear it, but I do bear it, because I don't have a choice. What would not bearing it look like? Crying hysterically? Losing my mind? Staying in bed all day? Well, I'm not doing any of those things, so I am bearing it.

I've still got my swollen belly and period-like cramps. Today I've also had a light pinkish beige discharge. At first, I was pleased, thinking implantation bleeding, but now I'm worried it could be the start of my period, which is why I nearly can't bear it. It would be early for my period, but not unheard of.

Oh, and the other thing is, I have tingly nipples. Lots of things point to 'Yes', and today I'd almost convinced myself that I must be pregnant, and I felt really happy, but now with the discharge and period-like feelings, I don't know what to think. I wish I could stop thinking altogether.

We bought a First Response pregnancy test. It says you can do it up to six days before your period is due, so technically I could do it now, but I don't know if I dare. The clinic said not to test early, so that you're sure the result is accurate once you do it. It does say it's more accurate the closer you get, so perhaps we could hold out two more days and do it Saturday morning. Maybe I'll ring the clinic and ask if I'm allowed to do it early.

Oh, I nearly can't bear it. Argh! Argh! Bleugh! I don't know what that is … I can't express it. Am I finally going insane?

Tori Day - Author

RESOURCES

Amber Woodward struggled with infertility for a number of years (four to be exact) before welcoming her IVF baby into the world. She is the founder of The Preggers Kitchen where she blogs – a humourous and light-hearted website on battling infertility, that is full of positivity, action, food and laughter.

If you would like to connect with Amber:

Website: www.thepreggerskitchen.com

Instagram @thepreggerskitchen

Andreia Trigo (RN, BSc, and MSc), is the founder of inFertile Life, multi-awarded nurse consultant, coach, author and TEDx speaker. Combining her fourteen-year medical experience, CBT, NLP and her own eighteen-year infertility journey, she has developed unique strategies to help people undergoing similar challenges, and achieve their reproductive goals. The Enhanced Fertility Programme is helping people worldwide and has been awarded Best Innovation in Business 2018 and E-Business of 2018.

If you would like to connect with Andreia:

Website www.andreiatrigo.com

Instagram @infertile_life

Anya Sizer had two children through IVF and another through adoption. She trained as a counsellor and worked in a fertility clinic, and is the London regional organiser of Fertility Network UK, a national charity dedicated to helping people with fertility problems. She also runs support groups. She is very vocal that NHS hospitals should follow national guidelines regarding offering three cycles of IVF treatment to each couple.

If you would like to connect with Anya:

Twitter @SizerAnya

Becky Kearns is mum to three donor egg conceived daughters and is very open about her infertility story – early menopause, numerous IVF cycles and loss – in the hope that she can inspire and support others who need to consider donor eggs to have their family. She blogs about infertility and having donor conceived children and her hope is that by speaking openly, both IVF and donor conception within society will become much more open and an accepted way of starting a family.

If you want to connect with Becky:

Website www.definingmum.com

Instagram @definingmum

Blair Nelson is an infertility warrior who began her journey in 2018, after she and her husband found out they were facing a challenging genetic factor when they began trying to start their family. It was then they were told IVF was their only option. After their second transfer from their first round of treatment, Blair suffered a heart-breaking miscarriage that redefined her life. Ever since then, she has made it her mission to bring facts, tips, inspiration and most importantly, a voice to the topic of infertility. She found her refuge in this difficult time amongst women who have been there, and she wants to return the favor. Her Instagram account, Fab Fertility, has grown into a brand, podcast and blog. In addition to continuing to start a family (three rounds of IVF complete), Blair is working to develop courses and templates to supplement her other ventures to help women navigate their journey.

If you would like to connect with Blair:

Website www.fabfertility.com

Facebook fabfertility

Pinterest @Fab Fertility

Instagram @fabfertility

YouTube Fab Fertility and

iTunes podcast Fab Fertility

Cat Strawbridge had a seven-year infertility journey, that included IUI, IVF, ICSI and two miscarriages. On her fourth IVF cycle, she got pregnant with twins, but sadly lost one of the identical twins at ten weeks. She is all too familiar with the anxiety and stress of baby loss and being pregnant after infertility, which is why she hosts The Finally Pregnant podcast. She is active on her personal Instagram account @tryingyears and is the 'Cat' half of Instagram account @itscatandalice, (the 'Alice' half is @thisisalicerose). Amongst other things Cat and Alice host Live Your Life: Fertility events – which include talks by health and wellbeing experts and people talking about their own fertility experiences. This offers the opportunity to connect with others who have similar situations to your own, plus there are goody bags and much more. Check out www.catandalice.com which has a global TTC meet up calendar as well as details of upcoming events.

If you would like to connect with Cat:

Website www.catstrawbridge.com,

Instagram @tryingyears

Diane Chandler is the author of Moondance, a novel about a couple struggling through the emotional and physical onslaught of fertility treatment. Diane herself underwent seven IVF cycles and she is one of the lucky ones who got there – her daughter is now sixteen.

If you would like to connect with Diane:

Website www.dianechandlerauthor.com

Twitter @DChandlerauthor

Facebook dianechandlerauthor

Dr Deborah Simmons had her own infertility journey before becoming the mother of two premature babies. She has provided specialized counseling for infertility-related trauma and pregnancy loss for more than twenty years. She works with fertility clinics, OB/GYN clinics, surrogacy agencies, and egg donor agencies around the United States. She provides psychoeducation to all who seek to be parents, whether this is by using IUIs, IVF, donor eggs, donor sperm, donor embryos, or gestational surrogacy. She offers clinical hypnosis, EMDR, cognitive behavioral therapy, couple's therapy, and energy work. She is also working in the area of fertility preservation with women who have been diagnosed with cancer and with transgender men and women who wish to be parents.

If you would like to connect with Dr Simmons:

Website www.partnersinfertility.net

Email drsimmons@partnersinfertility.net

Instagram @partners_in_fertility

Twitter @partnersinfert

Facebook partnersinfert

Dr Emma Brodzinski is a therapist and fertility coach. After her own fertility journey, she decided to use her skills as an expressive arts therapist and an academic researcher, alongside her experiences as a fertility patient, to support other women. She now delivers group courses as well as working one to one with clients and runs the 'IVF Got This' Facebook group and

The Pineapple Book Club.

If you would like to connect with Emma:

Website www.emmabrodzinski.com

Facebook emmabrodzinski

Instagram @emmabrodzinski

Pinterest @dremmabrodzinksi

FertilitySmarts was created by two women for whom getting pregnant was much more involved than they initially thought. They were surprised by the process it took to get there – including the inner workings of their bodies! But, when it came time to seek out more information about fertility options, all they found were sites full of useless gender quizzes and attempts at selling 'magic beans'.

What they were looking for was an evidence-based website about fertility, that broke down information in a helpful, easy-to-digest manner. This is exactly what they hope FertilitySmarts can be for you. Along with a dash of humor and a whole heap of compassion, they aim to provide information on everything to do with getting pregnant, and help you get smart about your fertility.

If you would like to connect with FertilitySmarts:

Website www.Fertilitysmarts.com

Facebook, Pinterest, Twitter and Instagram @fertilitysmarts

Jackie Figueras, MSN-Ed, RN, CPC, and Certified Fertility Coach, is a passionate and accomplished registered nurse, educator, and fertility support coach. Jackie received her training as a professional certified coach at the Institute for Professional Excellence in Coaching and has utilized these skills in her leadership role and with her personal coaching business. Her unique combination of being a nurse, an educator, a coach, and a patient who struggled with fertility issues, allow her to connect with her clients and provide engaging and interactive programs that set her apart from other communication specialists and fertility coaches. Struggling with fertility issues for years and having four consecutive miscarriages, including her daughters' twin, has created a deeper passion to change healthcare and the fertility journey for many women. She truly understands the impact stress can have on your physical, mental and emotional health and is dedicated to helping guide women on their own journeys to find more balance and peace.

If you would like to connect with Jackie;

Email jackie@thesupportivemama.com

Website www.thesupportivemama.com

Instagram @thesupportivemama

Facebook The Supportive Mama

Jessica Hepburn is one of the UK's leading patient voices on fertility, infertility, the science of making babies and modern families. Having been through eleven rounds of IVF, she understands what it's like to struggle to create the family you long for. She is the founder of Fertility Fest, the arts festival dedicated to fertility, as well as the author of The Pursuit of Motherhood and 21 Miles. She has also swum the English Channel, ran the London Marathon and climbed Kilamanjaro, Island Peak in Nepal, and Aconcagua, with more climbs planned.

If you would like to connect with Jessica:

Website www.jessicahepburn.com

Facebook jessicahepburnauthor

Twitter @jessicapursuit

Instagram @fertilityfest

Justine Bold has personal experience of infertility as she had a twelve year journey to motherhood, finally becoming a mum to twin boys in her forties. She has written articles on infertility and edited a book entitled: Integrated Approaches to Infertility, IVF and Recurrent Miscarriage that was published in 2016. She's also co-written a book on mental health that was published in 2019. She works as a University Lecturer and has research interests in lifestyle and nutrition and their links to health problems, such as endometriosis and polycystic ovarian syndrome.

If you would like to connect with Justine:

Twitter @justineboldfood

Instagram @justinebold

Website www.worcester.ac.uk/about/profiles/justine-bold

Justine Hankin has been named by The Daily Telegraph, The Guardian, Harper's Bazaar and The Culture Trip as one of the Top ten Acupuncture practitioners in the UK. Justine is a registered acupuncturist and fertility and women's health expert, and her expertise was included in the book The Stork Club by Imogen Edwards-Jones.

If you would like to connect with Justine:

Website www.justinehankin.co.uk

Facebook justinehankinacupuncture

Instagram @justinerhankin

Twitter @justinehankin

Kate Davies, RN, BSc(Hons), FP Cert, Fertility Nurse Consultant, has over twenty years' experience in fertility and women's health. She has also undertaken specialist training in PCOS, and has helped hundreds of women control their symptoms and go on to conceive. She is a qualified Fertility

Coach and offers her patients much needed emotional support as well as clinical advice. She is also a co-host, with Natalie (@ fertilitypoddy) on Talk Fertility, UK Health Radio – a weekly show discussing the wide range of issues affecting fertility.

If you would like to connect with Kate:

Instagram @your_fertility_journey

Website www.yourfertilityjourney.com

Email Kate@yourfertilityjourney.com

Facebook YourFertilityJourney

Twitter @fertjourney

Pinterest @yourfertilityjourney

Talk Fertility: www.ukhealthradio.com/blog/program/talk-fertility/

Lisa Attfield had her own eight-year fertility journey, before having her first child through IVF. She devised her own fertility yoga programme and used it before and during her fertility treatment to keep calm and positive.

If you would like to connect with Lisa:

Website www.fertilityyoga.co.uk

Twitter @FertilityYogaUK

Facebook Fertility-Yoga

Monica Bivas went through multiple IVF treatments – including the stillbirth of her second daughter – but was determined to try one last time. This time, however, she decided to approach her treatment with mindfulness and positivity which resulted in the birth of her third daughter. She now helps her tribe consciously direct their IVF experience by managing their emotions, shifting their mindsets, and preparing for the ultimate outcome of treatment – a precious baby. She is a regular contributor to the Huffington Post, and has published The IVF Planner, a journal and guide for women undergoing fertility treatment, and has another book forthcoming about her life-changing experience with IVF treatment. She is married to her amazing Israeli husband, Shai, whom she considers her best friend, and has two daughters and one step-daughter. Although born in Colombia, she is deeply in love with her home in Long Island, New York. When not supporting her IVF tribe, she fully immerses herself in being a hands-on mom, and a must in her life is a weekly date with her husband doing one of her favorite activities: dancing.

If you would like to connect with Monica:

Website www.monicabivas.com

Facebook monicabivasIVFcoach

Facebook Group theivfjourney

Twitter @MonicaBivas

Instagram @monicabivas

Pinterest @monicabivasivfcoach

Linkedin monicabivas

Mrs Meaks or Kate, lives in Surrey, UK, with her husband, Phil, and their son, Austin. Since Austin was born, she has been a stay at home mum whilst also continuing to have fertility treatment for another child. She is passionate about raising awareness of infertility and baby loss within the amazing TTC community, and she does this by being active on Instagram and her blog.

If you would like to connect with Kate,

Instagram @mrskmeaks

Blog www.mrsmeaks.com

Natalie Silverman had her own fertility journey and is the founder and host of the brilliant Fertility Podcast, where she aims to empower women and men trying to start or complete their families with expert interviews and real-life stories. She is also a co-host, with Kate (@your_fertility_journey) on Talk Fertility, UK Health Radio, a weekly show discussing the wide range of issues affecting fertility.

If you would like to connect with Natalie:

Instagram and Twitter @fertilitypoddy

Website www.thefertilitypodcast.com

Talk Fertility: www.ukhealthradio.com/blog/program/talk-fertility/

Nicola Salmon is a fat-positive and feminist fertility coach. She advocates for change in how fat women are treated on their fertility journey. She supports fat women – and others with disordered eating who are struggling to get pregnant – to find peace with their body, and find their own version of health to finally escape the yo-yo dieting cycle. For more information download The Fat Girl's Guide to Getting Pregnant @

www.nicolasalmon.co.uk/fat-girls-guide-getting-pregnant/

If you would like to connect with Nicola:

Instagram @fatpositivefertility

Website www.nicolasalmon.co.uk

Rachel Cathan is the author of the book: 336 Hours – a diary of one woman's battle through infertility and IVF during her five-year quest for motherhood. The story is set within the pressure cooker of the narrator's third, and supposedly final, IVF treatment. Rachel is also a fertility counsellor.

If you would like to connect with Rachel:

Website www.Rachelcathan.co.uk

Facebook 336hours

Twitter @rachelcathan

Sandra Bateman Reg MBACP (Accred) Reg MNFS Sen Accred Bio, is a Senior Fertility Counsellor and has been practicing in reproductive health for over twelve years in both private and NHS clinics. Sandra is an Accredited Member of the British Association for Counselling and Psychotherapy MBACP (Accred), and is the Chief Executive of the National Fertility Society and abides by their code of ethics. She is dedicated to educating and supporting patients through psychological and emotional wellbeing relating to reproductive health before, during and after IVF.

If you would like to connect with Sandra:

Email Sandra.bateman@nationalfertilitysociety.co.uk

Facebook @nationalfertilitysociety

Twitter @FERTILITYSOC

Instagram @national_fertility_society

Sophie Martin is a Registered Midwife, and infertility and baby loss advocate. Currently navigating the bumpy road of IVF, whilst also honouring the memory of her twin sons Cecil & Wilfred, after their very premature birth and death. She is dedicated to celebrating the power of women, and acknowledging how important it is to support other women on their journeys to motherhood.

If you would like to connect with Sophie:

Instagram @the.infertile.midwife

Tori Day, author of the book: Warrior: Battling infertility – Staying Sane While Trying to Conceive. Tori had her own rollercoaster infertility journey; 'Warrior' is her first book as an Indie author.

If you want to connect with Tori:

Twitter @ToriDayWrite

Thank you for reading

Would you like to help others as they negotiate their TWW? You can by leaving a review about this book on the online store you purchased it from.

How great is that?!

Sheila Lamb

Printed in Great Britain
by Amazon

79994586R00066